Dr. Gillian McKeith's
Living Food for Health

12 Natural Superfoods to Transform Your Health

DR. GILLIAN MCKEITH

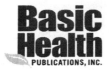

Basic Health
PUBLICATIONS, INC.

The information contained in this book is based upon the research and personal and professional experiences of the author. It is not intended as a substitute for consulting with your physician or other healthcare provider. Any attempt to diagnose and treat an illness should be done under the direction of a healthcare professional.

The publisher does not advocate the use of any particular healthcare protocol but believes the information in this book should be available to the public. The publisher and author are not responsible for any adverse effects or consequences resulting from the use of the suggestions, preparations, or procedures discussed in this book. Should the reader have any questions concerning the appropriateness of any procedures or preparation mentioned, the author and the publisher strongly suggest consulting a professional healthcare advisor.

Basic Health Publications, Inc.
28812 Top of the World Drive • Laguna Beach, CA 92651
949-715-7327 • www.basichealthpub.com

Published by arrangement with Judy Piatkus (Publishers) Limited, London, England

Library of Congress Cataloging-in-Publication Data

McKeith, Gillian.
    Dr. Gillian McKeith's living food for health : 12 natural superfoods
to transform your health.
      p. cm.
    ISBN-13: 978-1-59120-122-9
    ISBN-10: 1-59120-122-5
  1. Raw food diet. I. Title: Doctor Gillian McKeith's living food for
health. II. Title: Living food for health. III. Title.

    RM237.5.M355   2004
    613.2'6—dc22
                                              2004015400

Printed in the United States of America

10   9   8   7   6   5   4   3   2

CONTENTS

To my Auntie Rita who impressed upon me the importance of helping others to help themselves.

Hugs and kisses to my mum, dad, and wee daughter who hold that special place in my heart. Thank you so much for everything.

I am forever grateful to Marian Moore for sharing with me her gift of healing.

My gratitude extends to Paula Bartimeus, Jane Last, Pauline Norton, Anna Janschke, and Rachel Winning for their assistance. A special thank you to Badiene who introduced me to sprouts (not Brussels). My warmest appreciation to Ken Townson for his great photography work.

Special thanks to Doug and Eloise for their enlightenment and wisdom.

All my love to Howard to whom I am deeply grateful for his special words, editing, continual support, and encouragement. Howard, you introduced me to the field of natural health and, as a result, changed my life. Your inspiration fills me with enthusiasm, making me feel that anything is possible.

My dream is to share my experiences and information with anyone who will listen, perhaps sending them on a path to an even better quality of life and level of wellness. Together, I feel this mission will be realized.

1.

HOW LIVING FOODS CAN CHANGE YOUR LIFE

FIFTEEN YEARS AGO I WAS VERY ILL. I suffered with chronic fatigue, facial and stomach pains, gas, bloating, indigestion, continuous nausea, allergies, debilitating premenstrual tension, and a severely excruciating migraine that would not leave me. I would lie in bed most of each day. Yet I was cohosting the radio show *Healthline Across America* from New York, and interviewing experts and special guests about natural health. I loved that show so much that I dragged myself out of bed, drove to the studio to do the show, and quickly returned home just to get back into bed. Imagine the irony of it: a young girl hosting a national health radio show who is exhausted, sickly, and sleeps most of the time!

MOLDS AND MIRACLES

When my symptoms worsened, I started on the medical establishment "roller coaster." I visited dozens of specialists, each one prescribing more drugs than the previous one. I became even more debilitated. Finally, I met a brain surgeon who suspected that I had a life-threatening brain tumor. The doctor wanted me in the hospital as soon as possible for a brain scan. Strangely enough, my own brother was dating a girl with a brain tumor, and she had the same symptoms as me!

I prepared myself for death. I cherished every waking moment, every blade of grass. I smelled every rose and absorbed all aromas. I tried to convince myself that I might have to accept the fate of no children, no husband, dying young.

Luckily, the next day a spiritual energy healer was the special guest on the radio show. Afterward I asked her if she would work on me. With just a simple touch, she shifted the pain of my migraine for the first time in months. She told me that I did not have a brain tumor at all, and there was absolutely no need to go for the brain scan. Instead, she insisted that I be tested for severe allergies to yeast and molds. Reluctantly, I complied; and sure enough, she was right. Biochemical tests revealed that I was suffering from a rampant overgrowth of yeast in my blood, now known as *Candida albicans*. I was also diagnosed with severe allergy to molds.

I then spent years reeducating and retraining myself, earning a Ph.D. in clinical nutrition, and embarking upon a whole new adventure to find the path to perfect health. Ultimately, I worked for more than ten years in America researching the "superfoods"—what I now refer to as "living foods." Then about seven years ago, I returned to my native land to establish the McKeith Clinic in London.

HOW THIS BOOK CAN GET YOU ON THE PATH TO HEALTH

Category 1: Most People

As a clinical nutritionist, I help people to feel and look really well. That's my job. These are the people I call the *Category 1 patients,* who probably make up the vast majority of the general population. This category consists of people who just want to feel healthier, rejuvenated, and revitalized. There may not be anything wrong with them, except they just want to feel the best that they can. Sometimes, though, these people may have those little nagging complaints with which we can all relate. For example, "I'm tired," "I'm exhausted," "I get colds too easily," "my tummy feels bloated," "I have too much gas and flatulence," "I need to lose weight," "I don't move my bowels very well," "at that time of the month, my menstrual cramps are so painful," and so on. These are the kinds of problems that, at some point, we all experience—some more than others, though. Yet these problems are certainly not insurmountable nor irreparable. In fact, these patients often experience the best results from my program.

For example, I'm currently working with a thirty-two-year-old woman who came to me several months ago "just to lose a bit of weight," in her words. Not only has she lost the weight (approximately 14 pounds so far), but her high blood pressure has normalized; her cholesterol is now low; she no longer craves chocolate like before; her menstrual pains and other related symptoms have disappeared; biochemical tests now reveal that she is no longer deficient in minerals; she says that she feels "fabulous and energized." If I may say so myself, she actually looks much younger—improved skin tone, stronger nails, thicker hair, clearer eyes, and no dark circles under the eyes either. And best of all perhaps, she finally has become pregnant—something she had been attempting for some time.

This can definitely be you as well: feeling healthier, stronger, and looking better too. I see this every day at the clinic. My goal is to get you to this point. Once you embark upon my Living Food Program, you will feel and look so much better. So this book is for everyone who may not have specific health problems, but just wants to feel that much better. And I will help you get there.

Category 2: Everyone Else

As a clinical nutritionist and director of the McKeith Clinic, I have also successfully worked with just about every imaginable specific disease, illness, and malady that you could think of: constipation, premenstrual tension, headaches, depression, high blood pressure, high cholesterol, heart disease, insomnia, chronic fatigue, indigestion, immune dysfunction, multiple sclerosis, diabetes, hypoglycemia, infertility, irritable bowel syndrome, parasites, just to name a few. I'm not saying that I have a 100 percent success rate, but it's pretty close for those people who do exactly what I tell them. If you follow my program religiously, I am certain that most of your health complaints will disappear. It's not a question of ego (although some may beg to differ); I'm simply reporting to you the general results of my patients' treatment.

For instance, I often think about this one patient, the president of an international MS society in Europe. She arrived at my clinic basically crippled from multiple sclerosis: terrible bowel problems, constipation, shakiness, tremors, visual blackouts, numbness, and a walking stick for mobility. After about ten months on my Living Food Program, this MS patient no longer displayed these symptoms of the disease; and she no longer needed a walking stick either. I call this case one of the *Category 2 patients:* these are people who have specific diagnosed illnesses and we work on getting them well.

Category 3: Peak Performers

Finally, there are the *Category 3 patients.* These are people who want to perform at a much greater level. For example, one lady came to me at the age of forty-nine telling me that she wanted to run the London marathon! She had been a top runner thirty years previously, but hadn't really run since then. It was now up to me to whip her into nutritional shape so her dream could be realized. Lo and behold, several months later, she was running the marathon at the age of fifty! I can't say that she won the marathon; I actually wish that I could, because wouldn't that be a great testament to my program? But in the end, she finished in the top half, which I still think is rather amazing. These Category 3 patients also include a world-class boxer, an Olympic athlete, several well-known soccer players, and two very famous tennis players, who have all consulted with me in order to reach peak performances. I'm sure you can imagine their faces, especially the soccer players' (who love their beer, their french fries, and their wild nights out), when I come along and tell these spirited athletes that their fun will now come from a whole new way of life. Although I have found most professional athletes quite motivated, soccer players are not so easy. But once again, those who follow the program achieve fantastic results and top performance. My Olympic athlete has indicated that he might not be in the Olympics if it were not for the Living Food Program. I'm not saying that you will become an Olympic athlete if you adopt my program, but you never know!

The Way Forward

My patients are numerous and varied, and sing my praises only because of the results they get. It's not me doing it for them, please understand. They do it for themselves. As I tell my own patients, "I only show you the way. The rest is up to you." Once I give you the information, however, it becomes a much easier situation. I can assure you that if you do what I tell you, you will achieve favorable, often incredible results! My patients are the proof. And there are many of them for this good reason. I have consulted with movie stars, TV stars, radio stars, as well as world leaders, Royal family members, an internationally known artist, and presidents of some of the largest companies, not to mention taxi drivers, accountants, lawyers, teachers, students, housewives, plumbers, electricians, nurses, doctors, and even scientists. They all get the results, usually way beyond their expectations. I have patients who travel to the clinic from virtually every country of the world. And because there is an official waiting list with more than 900 names of patients who want to see me (as of 2000), I have recently (and unfortunately) had to halt scheduling these new patients. I can only now, for the most part, see current patients.

Therefore, please don't be offended if you call my office and they tell you there are no new patients being accepted for two years! First, as I have explained, I really cannot see new patients. Second, you can learn all the secrets from this book. Third, I am on a divine mission to share this essential information with as many people as possible for the good of civilization. In the time I could consult with just one patient, I can "talk" with millions of people via the media—through this book, television, radio, the Internet. I believe that the spiritual purpose of our lives is to *share,* not to just receive for oneself alone. Thus, I have made a commitment to myself, to my patients, and to my readers, that I will do everything possible to share my information with whomever will listen. In keeping with this commitment, I regularly appear on television in both the United States (for instance, *The Joan Rivers Show*) and the United Kingdom. I cohosted and produced the *Healthline Across America* radio show, one of America's most provocative and informative health programs. And I continue every day to research, test, and write furiously so that you may benefit.

Whether you want to

1. simply feel and look rejuvenated and revitalized,

2. heal a specific health problem, or

3. reach new heights,

this book can help you immensely and forever. The benefits of my Living Food Program have been achieved by thousands of people worldwide of all ages and walks of life and both genders. And now you too may obtain these extraordinary results. Sometimes even by adopting some subtle measures, people experience enormous long-term changes to their lives. I see it every day, and I know you can do it too.

THE BENEFITS OF LIVING FOODS

The benefits from my Living Food Program can be immense. In this book, you will learn all about these living foods, and specifically which foods can boost energy, strengthen blood, nourish the organs, and revitalize the cells. These are the very foods that healed me and now keep me strong. These living foods include live growing sprouts, supergrains such as millet or quinoa, seeds, sea vegetables (seaweeds), essential fatty acids, barley grass and other plants and herbs, along with wild blue-green algae. I ate these living foods every day, and this was the only way I could have recovered from my illnesses. But now I eat these living foods for vitality, well-being, and vigor.

Living foods increase vitality, strengthen the immune system, regulate weight, and slow down the aging process. They are packed with vitamins and minerals, have adequate protein, and are low in fat. They're rich in slow-releasing carbohydrates, which boost energy; and because living foods generally have a high fluid content, it makes them ideal for detoxifying the system. They're also rich in fiber. Soluble fiber lowers blood fat levels and removes heavy metals such as lead and cadmium from the body.

But the truly remarkable element of living foods, especially *raw* living foods, are *enzymes*. Enzymes are the key to proper food absorption, released as soon as we start to chew. All our physical processes depend on enzymes as well. Enzymes are the essential catalysts of all the chemical reactions in our bodies, without them we would cease to function or exist. Enzymes spark digestion, detoxification, immunity, and all other metabolic and regenerative processes. The quality of our enzymes is reflected in the vitality of our own energy levels and life force.

What Are Enzymes?

Enzymes, occurring in all living organisms, are protein molecules that digest our food, making food small enough to pass through the minute pores of the intestines into the blood. They are like the body's labor force. In addition to digesting food, enzymes also destroy toxins, break down fats and cellulose, and metabolize starch and proteins. Scientists have identified more than 2,500 different enzymes in the human body.[1] Enzymes are involved in every biochemical and physiological function. Everything we do as a living creature requires enzymes. All life processes are made up of a complex web of chemical reactions referred to as *metabolism*. Enzymes are the very catalysts that make metabolism happen. So the catalyst, or the enzymes in the case of humans, is the biochemical material that initiates the necessary chemical reactions to make life possible.

Therefore, without enzymes, we would cease to exist. And with low enzyme activity, we can experience some pretty devastating conditions. Dr. Anthony Cichoke in his book *Enzymes & Enzyme Therapy* makes no bones about the importance of enzymes to the human species. He states that our bodies depend on enzymes to think, breathe, walk, talk, digest food, and function at optimum capacity. For the body to operate at its peak, fight off illness, and repair injured cells, enzymes need to be plentiful and vital. Enzymes renew, defend, and support our systems.[2] Interestingly enough, there is a medical doctor in New York City, Nicholas Gonzales, M.D., whom I have interviewed a few times on the radio. Dr. Gonzales reported many significant case studies, using primarily megadoses of enzymes and enzyme-rich foods, in successfully treating cancer and other degenerative diseases.

So as you can imagine, the level of enzyme content within our foods is a more than critical issue. The strength of enzyme function is essential for the strength of our health and well-being. At the McKeith Clinic, we administer a series of biochemical tests to evaluate enzyme activity. The greatest problem I have seen with patients suffering from low enzyme activity has to do with gastrointestinal disorders: indigestion, malabsorption, heartburn, burping, flatulence, bloating, cramps, constipation, irritable bowel syndrome, and chronic fatigue. When the enzyme activity is restored, these disorders are almost always eradicated.

There are three basic classifications of enzymes:

1. *Metabolic enzymes,* which direct our bodies; they act as catalysts in building bone, repairing tissue, regulating metabolism, talking, breathing, reproduction, hearing, and every muscle movement. These metabolic enzymes occur naturally within our bodies' biochemistry. Yet as we age, the metabolic enzyme activity lessens.

2. *Digestive enzymes* are required in digesting food; these enzymes break down proteins, carbohydrates, and fats from food. The digestive enzymes are also responsible for extracting, assimilating, metabolizing, and absorbing nutrients, vitamins, and minerals.

3. *Food enzymes* help the digestive process. They must come from the foods

we eat. All live raw foods—namely raw fruits, raw vegetables, raw seeds, raw nuts, certain key superfoods, and especially live sprouts—are the sources for food enzymes.

Raw meats and raw fish also contain enzymes, but I absolutely forbid the eating of raw meats and raw fish for a host of pathogenic and parasitic reasons, to which I do not have the time or space to devote in this book. Meat or fish should be cooked thoroughly. Thus, when I refer to "raw living foods," for the purpose of this book, I am talking about *non*-animal-based foods only. Nonetheless, there are enough non-animal-based raw living foods bounding with enzymes for us to ignore the animal-based ones.

From my clinical experience, I have found that low enzyme activity is perhaps the most prevalent problem among modern Western people today. A fast-track, upwardly mobile life, accompanied by fast food, has translated into a population that is virtually devoid of digestive enzymes. The implications are far-reaching and serious, yet reversible and correctable. And my job here is to reverse and correct the bad, and then to get you on the good path—rejuvenation, revitalization, total well-being, perfect health. It's all within our grasp.

TAKE THE ENZYME EXAM

Do you recognize yourself?

If you suffer from one or more of the following symptoms, then you may need more ENZYME-RICH FOOD in your diet.

❏ Do you eat processed foods, fast foods, microwaved foods, "boil in the bag" type foods three or more times a week?

❏ Is your diet high in refined sugar?

❏ Do you eat cooked foods more than three times a week?

❏ Is your diet low in raw fruits and vegetables?

❏ Do you drink alcohol regularly?

❏ Do you drink coffee or caffeinated tea on a daily basis?

❏ Do you eat fast? (Food needs to be chewed thoroughly; your stomach doesn't have teeth.)

❑ Do you drink carbonated beverages more than three times a week?

❑ Do you feel tired after you eat?

❑ Are you constipated?

  a) ❑ bowels move only once a day when eating three meals daily

  b) ❑ bowels move less than once a day

  c) ❑ bowel movements are difficult

  d) ❑ you produce "rabbit droppings"

❑ Do you have diarrhea regularly? Itchy anus?

For the next couple of questions you will need to look at your stools.

❑ Are your stools filled with mucus?

❑ Do you produce stools that just won't flush (that is, keep floating)?

❑ Do you see undigested food in your stools?

Take a look at your nails.

❑ Do you have ridges on your nails?

❑ Do you have white spots on your nails?

Find a mirror and stick out your tongue.

❑ Is there a line running down the middle of your tongue?

❑ Are there teeth marks around the sides of your tongue (that is, scalloped edging)?

❑ Are there any cracks on your tongue?

Do you suffer from any of the following?

❑ psoriasis

❑ eczema

❑ hives

❑ Do you suffer from any allergies?

❏ Do you have a debilitating illness?

❏ Do you smoke? Shame on you!

❏ Are you a *new* parent?

❏ Are you under stress?

❏ Do you experience excessive hair loss?

If you answered "yes" to any of the first seven questions, please add more *living* foods into your diet.

If you exhibit one to eight of the above symptoms, you need to increase the amount of enzyme-rich foods.

If you exhibit nine to sixteen of the above symptoms, you need to increase your supply of enzyme-rich foods. You may need to take a digestive enzyme with all cooked meals. Eat more raw foods and sprouts. Include mineral-rich foods in your diet.

If you exhibit seventeen to twenty-five of the above symptoms, you must dramatically increase the amount of enzyme-rich food in your diet. Eat more raw sprouts, fruits, and vegetables. Add other living foods into your life that are high in minerals. Take two digestive enzymes with every meal.

THE CLINICAL STUDIES

Now, as director of the McKeith Clinic in London, I can report key clinical research and case studies to support the efficacy of these living foods.

First, almost all of the patients who first come to consult me are eating "dead foods." As soon as we cook, boil, bake, fry, steam, or even freeze our foods, we destroy the active nutrients and the live enzymes. The enzymes are essential for

1. digesting foods,

2. extracting nutrients from the food,

3. dissolving fat,

4. reproduction,

5. scavenging free radicals.

Second, according to blood or sweat tests, 98 percent of the patients are deficient in one or more minerals when they initially visit the clinic. The danger is that a deficiency in even just one mineral can cause imbalances in many other minerals, vitamins, and amino acids—like a chain reaction or domino effect. And the vast majority of new patients come with tired or sluggish organs.

Third, most patients are either unable or unwilling to eat a diet of living raw foods. When I start telling people to grow sprouts, or to eat sea vegetables, seeds, plants, or herbs, they just look blank. So several years ago, I began to experiment with the dry powders of these living foods. Using a cold process to dry live sprouts and other living foods, these dry powders were then administered to patients at the clinic. In effect, I made it easy for them. My patients only needed to mix the powder in juice, water, or soups. I just wanted to get living foods into their bodies somehow, and this was the only way it seemed to work on a practical level.

Ultimately, however, I would prefer that people use real living foods: it would be best to grow your own sprouts, use sea vegetables whenever possible, and eat lots of fresh (organic) vegetables, fruits, seeds, legumes, nuts, herbs, and plants. Experience has taught me, however, that human nature often prevents people from being such goody-goodies; most may not have the time, the energy, the will, or the knowledge to eat so perfectly. Nonetheless, the clinical results of patients using the living food powder were astounding. These patients who regularly ate the living superfoods, or at least my living food powders, saw major biochemical changes take place via blood, sweat, stool, and even urine tests.

Case Study: Female, 28, Attorney

In one clinical case, for example, a woman from Surrey suffered from severe zinc deficiency, according to blood and sweat tests. Zinc deficiency may lead to infertility and immune dysfunction. When the patient was prescribed zinc lozenges, zinc capsules, and even liquid zinc, the deficiency did not correct itself. But when she used a diet of living foods plus additional algae for approximately two months, her zinc levels normalized: she was no longer deficient in zinc.

She also reported greater sexual desire, dramatically improved energy levels, and the halting of a constant cycle of colds and influenza. Her immune system was significantly enhanced and her monthly symptoms of premenstrual tension had vanished. During the period of the zinc deficiency, she was unable to conceive after months of trying. But shortly after her zinc level normalized, she became pregnant. I can now report that she recently gave birth to a very healthy baby.

Case Study: Male, 46, Banker

Another patient, who worked in the city of London, came to me with horrendous bloating, gas, indigestion, malabsorption, constipation, and frequent mood swings. Biochemical tests revealed a severe magnesium deficiency, amino acid imbalance, and sluggish liver. After just five weeks on the living foods, accompanied by a series of colonic treatments, his mineral and amino acid levels normalized. Most important, his symptoms disappeared. He reported: "increased energy levels, endurance, stamina, improved memory and elevated mood, better focus at work, more concentration, and a feeling of satisfaction that I never felt before."

Clinically Significant

The kinds of excellent results shown in these case studies were typical, and thus too numerous and too clinically significant to ignore. In almost every case, nutritional deficiencies were corrected and mineral, vitamin, and amino acid levels came into perfect balance. Patients inevitably reported major shifts in health: increased stamina and energy levels, improved immunity, and even enhanced mental clarity, memory, and organ response. Living foods, in essence, feed the cells, nourish the organs, tone the blood, regulate the bowels, strengthen muscle tissue, and ultimately boost immunity.

The Physiology

Here's how it works physiologically. Living foods are active live superfoods. These superfoods include live sprouted grains, which have the greatest level of nutritional and bioavailable vitality. Living sprouts are at the highest stage of growth, and thus provide the most usable and digestible nutrients and live enzymes. Because the body recognizes the nutrients from live food, the absorption, metabolism, and assimilation rates are far better.

Conversely, as soon as foods are cooked (especially at high heat), frozen, or canned, you now know that they lose their nutrient content. Living foods, on the other hand, may contain on average 85 percent more bioavailable nutrient value.

Our Energy Battery: The Spleen

Furthermore, living foods nourish all the organs, especially the endocrine system, pancreas, liver, kidneys, and most of all, the spleen. In my clinical practice, I have found that the single most important factor in achieving perfect health is directly dependent upon the strength and vitality of the internal organs. When the organs are in optimum form and working to maximum capacity, then everything else works optimally too.

The implications of sluggish organs are far-reaching. Sluggish or tired organs could cause us to become tired, chronically fatigued, irritable, con-stipated, confused, angry, stressed, depressed, violent, diseased, or worse. Sluggish organs translate into an even more sluggish you, especially since each organ is dependent on other organs for life support. On the other hand, when we strengthen our key organs, we become calmer, more focused, energized, nourished, happier, and healthier overall—with a stronger immune system. For example, the spleen is essential in digesting, assimilating, and transporting nutrients to the blood. If the spleen is not in perfect order, it becomes difficult (sometimes impossible) to absorb vita-mins, minerals, or even amino acids properly; and the blood often becomes compromised as a result. Therefore, if you suffer from a tired spleen, it may not matter how many healthy supplement pills I prescribe; the truth is that a sluggish spleen inhibits absorption of nutrients. You could swallow bucketfuls of vitamin pills, yet not absorb an iota of good-ness from them—if the spleen is weak.

When we eat too many processed, preservative-laden, and over-cooked foods, we weaken our spleens. Seventy percent of new patients at the clinic have sluggish spleens, according to biochemical tests. Common indicators of this condition might include indigestion, burping, malabsorption, heartburn, bloating, flatulence, exhaustion, depression, or poor immunity. If you suffer from any of these symptoms, the chances are that you have a weak spleen. Weak spleens are the result of too much enzyme-deficient foods, mucus-producing foods (that is, too much dairy food and a poor diet), incorrect food combining, stress, and even giving birth. The spleen is the critical organ that regulates the number of red blood cells in circulation, destroys old red blood cells, and stores iron. The spleen releases many potent immune system-enhancing compounds into the blood.

Medical researcher, Stephen Gascoigne, emphasizes in the *Manual for Conventional Medicine* the importance of maintaining a strong spleen energy.[3] He states that if spleen energy is depleted for any reason, then the gastrointestinal function is compromised, resulting in an overproduction of mucus. This excess mucus collects in the organs and can cause all kinds of problems ranging from bowel disorders to Crohn's disease, ulcerative colitis, and even chronic bronchitis, if the mucus passes into the lungs. According to Dr. Gascoigne, excess mucus can even lodge in the skin, causing eczema.[4]

For those people living in a damp environment such as the United Kingdom, it is even more critical to strengthen the spleen with living foods in order to help build blood and immunity. The spleen is an organ that is weakened and aggravated by a damp environment. Damp moisture droplets and wet molecules can easily invade the body, precipitating a condition of damp, wet mucus internally. Damp drowns the spleen, choking its functions, collecting in the head, chest, stomach, joints, and organs.

In my own clinical practice, based in the great—yet damp—city of London, I have seen many more cases of weakened spleens than I have witnessed in other parts of the world. London seems to be full of people blowing noses with constant catarrh (inflammation of mucous membranes) and congestion. It is no wonder that we British are the most internationally traveled people in the world, especially to places with a bit of dry sun. Prolonged exposure to environmental damp (rain, drizzle, thick cloud cover, fog) can be a catalyst for making the body heavy, slow, and bloated. Conditions of indigestion; skin eruptions; heaviness in the limbs, legs, and head; lethargy; fullness in the stomach; bloating; loose stools; or diarrhea may result. However, damp mucus in the body can be caused not only by climatic conditions, but from external elements such as poor food choices, stress, and overload of chemical toxins as well. However, if the spleen and other organs are strong, then the body will not necessarily react or become weakened by a damp environment. In effect, it might not make any significant difference to your body when it rains for a week—if your health is in a strong state. Nonetheless, when my own patients start to eat spleen-strengthening foods and foods that resolve dampness, such as parsley, garlic, daikon, radishes, turnips, barley grass, adzuki beans, and algae, we then see a dramatic improvement. I tell my patients that environmental dampness can really only gain entry when the person is weak or under the weather. Even if a person is lucky enough to live in a dry environment, but eats a diet of dead, mucus-producing foods, that person can still suffer from a weak spleen and internal mucus.

Finally, healthy blood depends on a well-functioning digestive system. The spleen assists the stomach in the digestion process and, ultimately, in building the blood. In its operation, the spleen actually transports and transforms nutrients into usable energy, eventually producing healthier blood.

You Are What You Absorb

Therefore, if your spleen is compromised, you will be less able to absorb nutrients from foods or supplement pills. At the clinic, I have seen whole vitamin tablets expelled from the feces during colonic hydrotherapy treatments. These patients were simply not breaking down the vitamin pills, as they had weak spleens causing digestive ills. When I prescribed living foods to patients with digestion problems, we would see noticeable improvements in nutrient uptake as absorption, assimilation, and metabolism of vitamins and minerals dramatically improved. This was because of

1. the high level of live active enzymes in the living foods,

2. the active level of vitamins, minerals, and amino acids within the powder itself,

3. the nourishing effect of living foods on all the organs, especially the spleen. When the spleen is nourished, the digestion, assimilation, and absorption of nutrients improves significantly.

As I tell my own patients, in order to achieve perfect health, it's not what you ingest that counts; rather it's what you *absorb* that really matters. As you can imagine, therefore, I am not a nutritionist who is concerned with potencies and milligrams of vitamins. Some people may not absorb more than 5 or 10 percent of a conventional supplement pill. But when you obtain your nutrients from live foods with live enzymes, then your absorption of vitamins and minerals will be at maximum capacity.

Perfect Balance, Perfect Health

In the clinical trials with patients at my clinic, I used a living food powder that was perfectly and synergistically harmonized to provide a biochemical benefit to each organ and each meridian of the body. My husband says I'm obsessed with "balance" because I am astrologically a Libra, the sign of balanced judgment. I tell him it's because I'm committed to getting people well. I developed the living food powder (although I recommend people eat actual live foods) in perfect balance. In the West, we are always looking at the protein content, vitamins, minerals, enzymes, and so on of a food. Yet in the East, they consider the energetic quality a food provides the body and its subsequent effects on the whole *psychological* system after digestion. I try to balance both Western and Eastern medical and biochemical philosophies to create harmony. At the McKeith Clinic and in my own home food preparation, I also merge these two concepts. While considering the nutritional value of food, I recognize that various foods possess different energies and perform different actions in the body. Some foods warm us up; others cool us down. For example, if we only eat predominantly spicy foods, we need to bring balance by using cooling foods such as cucumber. If not, we will destroy our delicate internal balance of fluids.

This is not the same as hot or cold in terms of temperature. For example, we can include warming herbs, such as basil, ginger, or cinnamon, in a salad to warm us up. All cells and molecules, and therefore all foods too, maintain energetic qualities. Every organism and every food molecule delivers an energy or vibrational field. Once we understand these energy fields, we can better manipulate and balance our foods for medicinal purposes with great therapeutic impact.

I developed a combination living food powder for clinical purposes in a specific formulation, which would address the balancing of such energy fields. In effect, the powder contains certain foods that "warm" the body, while others "cool." Some foods moisturize, while others dry, and so on. This is the best way to eat—in perfect balance. For instance, the wild blue-green algae in the powder assists in "drying" damp conditions such as mucus, phlegm, and catarrh. Similarly, the live sprouted millet contained in the powder helps to "cool" the body, while the live sprouted quinoa helps to "warm" the body, while other ingredients moisturize.[5]

In addition, the millet sprouts specifically nourish the spleen. Millet is also an antifungal agent, high in iron, magnesium, and silicon, which builds cell tissue for healthy bones, hair, skin, nails, and teeth. Sprouted quinoa, a supergrain from the Americas, strengthens the kidneys. It is the most nutrient-dense grain with high levels of iron, vitamin E, and B complex. In its sprouted form, quinoa contains more calcium than milk and more usable protein than meat!

The flax works to lubricate the body with its high content of essential fatty acids. The essential fatty acids, which are contained in my living food powder, regulate the function of every organ, gland, and cell. These essential fatty acids, derived from the highest quality flax (linseed), sunflower, and the sea vegetable nori, are necessary for

1. building healthy blood,

2. nourishing the adrenal glands better to handle stress,

3. nutrifying the thyroid glands properly to manage weight control,

4. enhancing fertility,

5. preventing heart disease.

The green barley grass in the living food powder contains extraordinary amounts of SOD (superoxide dismutase), the key antioxidant enzyme helping to clear the cells of radiation, chemical pollutants, and other toxins. I included parsley because it actually contains more vitamin C than citrus fruit! Parsley also works on the spleen and liver. The powder also contains aloe vera, alfalfa, and the sea vegetable dulse.

The sweet herbal plant called stevia is included in the powder. This plant is twenty-five times sweeter than sugar, yet with none of the negative effects of regular sugars. Stevia is, in fact, not a sugar at all. I added this remarkable plant because it helps regulate blood sugar, as it suppresses the desire for sweets and lessens hunger cravings.

As a result, several overweight patients have reported weight loss and sustained weight control while using the living food powder. Although I do not recommend the powder as a meal replacement, I am currently consulting with an obese patient from Yorkshire who is using the powder and who has consistently lost seven pounds every month for the past four months, a total weight loss of just under 28 pounds. Several other patients have experienced significant weight loss or weight control.

The Most Advanced Nutritional Foundation

It has taken me a lifetime of clinical research, case studies, medical reports, and a labor of love to create the perfect living food combination— the ideal nutritional foundation, with the correct harmonizing balance for all tissues, organs, cells, and membranes of the human body. I am convinced that this is the most scientifically advanced formula to benefit the whole population. I feel blessed to be able to share my knowledge of living foods with everyone.

It is important to note that the super twelve ingredients discussed here are certainly not the total of all healthy live superfoods. It's just that these specific foods were most beneficial for healing and strengthening my patients and me. When taken together, for the purpose of counteracting cultural, climatic, and modern environmental issues, they nourish our organs, feed the cells, and revitalize the body. These combined foods have special synergistic interplay together. The only reason I mention the living food powder is because it was the powder on which the clinical case studies were based. I would have preferred that the trials be based on subjects eating actual real living foods, but the patients found it too difficult to stick to the necessary diet in the strict manner that I required. But when I prepared the living food powder myself for the patients to take home and use in water or juice, they were receptive, willing, and cooperative. In this way, I was able to track the clinical results more accurately.

My best advice to you, however, is to go with the actual real foods as much as possible. You can assume that any beneficial results achieved by the patients using the powder would pale in comparison to the results that you could achieve by eating the real thing. The balanced formulation of the twelve living foods, which are specifically tailored, healing, and strengthening to the modern Western population, include sprouted millet, sprouted quinoa, alfalfa, aloe vera, green barley grass, wild blue-green algae, flax, parsley leaves, the seaweeds nori and dulse, the stevia plant, and sunflower.

These are the superfoods, in the specific balance that ultimately healed me, then strengthened my organs, blood, and whole body. I now use these same living foods to heal, rejuvenate, and revitalize my own patients at the clinic. In the following chapters, I will outline each living food and its energetic balance so that you can fully understand the way they work and the relevant implications to your own health and well-being. Then we will look at dozens of other living foods as well.

THE SACRED 12

The following is a list of the 12 living foods that healed me, then revitalized, regenerated, and strengthened my cells, blood, and organs. These are the same superfoods that also work wonders for my patients at the clinic, in a balanced and harmonized combination. Now these living foods can work for you too:

1. Sprouted millet	7. Parsley
2. Sprouted quinoa	8. Dulse
3. Alfalfa	9. Nori
4. Aloe vera	10. Stevia
5. Green barley grass	11. Sunflower
6. Flax seeds	12. Wild blue-green algae

Although this makes up the sacred 12, the foundation of the key superfoods from which to start, we will explore many other living foods as well.

2.

SUPER SPROUTS
FOR SUPERHEALTH

NUTRITIONALLY:
bursting with enzymes, antioxidant enzymes, anti-aging
constituents, vitamins, trace minerals, amino acids, chlorophyll,
complete protein, fiber and pigments.

PHYSIOLOGICALLY:
support all organs.

BENEFITS:
improved digestion, vitality, energy; stronger, life-enhancing
protection against free radicals.

One of the greatest studies ever conducted in the field of natural health
was supervised by Dr. Edmond Bordeaux Szekely over a period of thirty-
three years, whereby he evaluated more than 120,000 people on the
experimental effects of eating raw live foods.[6] The health benefits to the
study groups, which he summarized, were unsurpassed as compared to
the control groups. Dr. Szekely concluded his lifetime of research by issu-
ing four very specific dietary food categorizations. The most malign category he called *bioacidic*. These are the destructive foods, those processed
with chemicals, preservatives, and irradiation, and are genetically modified. They degrade life functions.

The next category, perhaps not as negative as the first, is *biostatic*
foods. Nonetheless, biostatic foods do nothing to improve the living organism. This category refers to primarily cooked foods, or even foods that
are simply not fresh. Biostatic foods retard biochemical functions and
accelerate aging, according to Szekely.

Then there is the category of *bioactive* foods. This category refers to fresh raw fruits and vegetables, seeds, beans, legumes, and nuts. In effect, these are foods that sustain a healthy life force.

Finally, and most significantly, Dr. Szekely highlights the most important category he terms *biogenic* foods.[7] These are the most life-enhancing high-energy superfoods. They are alkaline-producing (as opposed to acid-forming) complete proteins, with chelated minerals, nucleic acids, vitamins, RNA, and DNA, and highest in active enzymes. Biogenic foods improve, revitalize, strengthen, regenerate, and enhance the human condition. This biogenic category consists of all sprouts.

WHAT ARE SPROUTS?

I'm not talking about Brussels sprouts here. Sprouts generally refer to the seeds of legumes or grains that have been germinated (usually without sunshine or soil) into baby plants within three to five days. These seeds or grains are then called sprouted, or grown into sprouts, and I'll explain how you can do this in your own kitchen on page 30.

Sprouting is the process of soaking, then germinating the seed, and finally eating the growing live sprouts. I have found that millet and quinoa sprouts can be used for the most exceptional therapeutic health benefits in energizing the mind, body, blood, and organs. Here is a list of what else may be sprouted:

- *The Seeds*—pumpkin, sunflower, sesame, alfalfa, mustard, fenugreek, radish, buckwheat, clover.

- *The Grains*—quinoa, millet, wheat, rye, maize, rice, corn, oats, barley, spelt, amaranth, kamut.

- *The Nuts*—almonds, cashews, hazelnuts, Brazil nuts, pine nuts, pecans, pistachios, walnuts, and so on.

- *The Pulses*—lentils, adzuki beans, kidney beans, navy beans, garbanzo beans (chickpeas), blackeye peas, soybeans, lima beans, mung beans, green peas.

Each sprouting seed is complete with the nutritional and microbiological energy and life force strong enough to create a full grown healthy plant. Once the seed is soaked in water, one of the necessary steps for sprouting, further beneficial elements develop. For example, the soaking process of a seed activates the release of additional enzymes, which otherwise would have been dormant.[8] The actual germination of the seed into a sprout represents the creation of a new plant. There can be no greater life energy than the creation of a new life force.[9] Upon germination, the seed rapidly absorbs water (from soaking) and swells to at least twice its original size. Simultaneously, the nutrient content swells too. The husk of the seed contains the embryo, which grows into both the root and the shoot.

Meanwhile, the endosperm and cotyledons (two inside halves) become the food supply for the growing plant. Enzymes, vitamins, minerals, amino acids, proteins, essential fatty acids, and other cofactors all dramatically increase during this process.

Finally, the germination process effectively predigests the seed, making its nutrients totally available for digestion and assimilation by us. For example, the explosive increase in enzymes converts starch into simple sugars, protein into freeform amino acids, and fats into essential fatty acids. This may explain the reason why certain beans or grains that ordinarily might cause sensitivities or allergic reactions for some people, generally do not do so when in a sprouted form. The predigestion process of germination renders these constituents bioavailable and perfectly assimilable to our bodies. The end result for us is a superfood with enormous levels of proteins, vitamins, minerals, trace minerals, chlorophyll pigments, and enzymes, which have all multiplied anywhere from 300 to 1,200 percent in the most easily digestible form.[10] By sprouting, we not only gain the benefits of the raw food, but also dramatically increase the nutrient content of these seeds and grains. Sprouts generally have far greater nutrient activity than all other raw foods because, in effect, the sprouts are still in the process of growing at the peak of life force.

The Nutrient Connection

Specifically, sprouts contain a high concentrate of antioxidant nutrients such as vitamins A, C, E, and B. Antioxidants protect against free radicals—unstable molecules that cause oxidation or aging, damaging cell tissue. Sprouts also contain all the trace minerals, including much needed selenium and zinc, plus bioflavonoids, all the freeform amino acids, antioxidant enzymes, especially superoxide dismutase (SOD), as well as chlorophyll and fiber. Sprouts release two anti-aging constituents—RNA and DNA (nucleic acids)—that are found only in living cells. The body also absorbs nutrients more efficiently from live sprouts, than say from nutrient supplements, because the body recognizes the sprouts as food. In particular, a study conducted at Yale University by Dr. Paul Barkholden found that B vitamins increased in sprouts by as much as 2,000 percent.[11] Biotin increases by as much as 50 percent, inositol 100 percent, pantothenic acid (B_5) 200 percent, pyridoxine (B_6) 500 percent, folic acid 600 percent, and both B_2 and B_{12} by as much as 2,000 percent. Even laetrile, known as the anti-cancer B_{17} nutrient, increased by 50 to 100 percent, depending upon the specific sprouted seeds.[12] A research study at the University of Pennsylvania (my alma mater) by Dr. Barry Mack reported a general overall average vitamin increase of more than 500 percent when seeds have sprouted.[13] D. C. Andrea of McGill University found that certain sprouts contain just about as much vitamin C as a glass of orange juice.[14] Dr. R. Bogart of the Kansas Agricultural Experimental Station measured more vitamin C content in sprouts than in certain melons and berries.[15]

Nucleic acids, the fundamental constituents required for cell growth and regeneration, increased by up to thirty times after sprouting seeds.[16] In addition to the enormous vitamin content, sprouts are the best source of trace minerals next to the sea vegetables dulse and nori, which I'll discuss later in Chapter 10. Most sprouts are extraordinarily high in calcium, magnesium, germanium, and iron, as well as selenium, manganese, chromium, zinc, and dozens more. The minerals in sprouts are chelated, which simply means that they are in a form far more digestible and absorbable by the human body.[17]

In one major study, researchers A. M. Maiser and A. Poljakoff-Mayber at Hebrew University found that sprouting decreases or eliminates the sometimes naturally occurring undesirable elements in foods, such as phosphates or a substance called phytin. Yet at the same time, according to this study, sprouts increase the level of desirable elements such as phosphorus, lecithin and phospholipids, which help assimilate and transport essential fatty acids, aiding fat metabolism, cholesterol and hormone regulation, brain function, and reproduction.[18]

The Protein Connection

The protein content of almost any seed also increased by 15 to 30 percent when sprouted, according to Elson Haas, M.D., in his book *Staying Healthy With Nutrition*.[19] Professor of Nutritional Biochemistry at University of Puget Sound, Dr. Jeffrey Bland showed that approximately six cups of sprouts could potentially supply the recommended daily nutritional intake for the average adult. Dr. Bland concluded that sprouts are a "more efficient, healthier (and certainly cheaper!) form of protein than the conventional animal or even other types of vegetable proteins."[20] Researchers at Purdue University, Department of Botany and Plant Pathology, found that germinated corn sprouts created high concentrations of two key amino acids, lysine and tryptophan, both building blocks for protein. The researchers concluded their study by stating that sprouts could provide high-quality protein nutritional foods for human consumption.[21]

In a different study, but at the same university, Dr. C. Y. Tsai found that sprouts in general maintain high levels of protein. In some cases, the protein concentration of certain sprouts was shown to be in excess of 25 percent of calories, which represents more protein than a standard beef steak (and in more digestible form too!).[22]

Finally, reaching back into scientific archives, I found that Dr. C. McCay of Cornell University was hired by the American government during World War II to find suitable protein alternatives to meat in the event of expected food shortages. After many months of research, Dr. McCay issued a report stating that the germination of sprouted seeds or beans could provide the protein requirements to the American population. At the time, several of Dr. McCay's articles and even recipes appeared in literature made available by the official U.S. Government Printing Office.[23] However, such food shortages never materialized in the United States. The literature and the subsequent campaign to educate Americans about sprouts was ultimately dropped a couple of years later. In fact, sprouts are higher in protein than most common lettuces, spinach, or other leafy green vegetables.

The Enzyme Connection

This now brings us back to those ever-critical enzymes. You now know the absolute importance of enzymes from Chapter 1. But it was Szekely, in his massive study of foods, who made the connection between enzymes and sprouts. To enhance health, we must eat living foods containing active enzymes. Sprouts are the ultimate living foods with the most abundant sources of such active enzymes. The activity of enzymes is at its peak during the germinating stage when a plant begins to sprout. Gabriel Cousens, M.D., in his book *Spiritual Nutrition,* points out that germinating and sprouting increase enzyme levels by six to twenty times, depending upon the specific plant.[24]

If our diet is lacking in enzymes, the food we eat moves far slower through the digestive tract and can literally rot, putrefy, and ferment in the intestines. The end result: toxins circulate in the body from the colon and from there into the bloodstream. These are seen as "foreign" invaders by the immune system, and the body must expend great amounts of energy removing them. This overexpenditure of energy leads to lethargy, exhaustion, chronic fatigue, and weakened immunity. When we fill our diet with high enzyme foods—specifically sprouts of all kinds—we can usually feel dramatic improvements to overall health and well-being.

I have one patient, a mother of five, who has indeed embarked upon a diet of mostly raw foods and loads of different sprouts. She has been coming to me for about three years, and on this living foods regimen for almost all that time. When she first started to consult with me, her cholesterol and blood pressure were high, where now both are correctly low. Her blood mineral levels are now delightfully high, whereas before they were severely and sadly deficient. She tells me now that she feels "absolutely fantastic," and begs at every office visit to take me out to lunch—to a living foods restaurant hopefully! Interestingly enough, this very busy mother actually looks much younger today than when she first came to me. The positive biochemical changes will not only manifest in laboratory tests, but the patient will feel and look so much better too.

One other note. My own sister-in-law frequents a raw living foods cleansing center in California about every four to six months. She goes to this warm, dry climate for about three weeks at a time, eating nothing but living foods, especially sprouts, and gets colonic hydrotherapy. All I can tell you is that each time she returns from this retreat, she looks fifteen or so years younger—at least. In fact, the last time she went to the Center, she came back with a boyfriend at least that many years her junior! I had better quit while I'm ahead and move on to our next topic, so that I don't fall out with my beloved sister-in-law. The point here, however, is that you, too, really can look physically so much younger, and perform better too. And by the way, my sister-in-law does look smashing.

The Immune Connection

Finally, to me, this is what it's all about: strengthening the immune system so we are better equipped to prevent and combat common colds and flu, illnesses, even dreaded diseases. Living foods help to keep the immune system strong. When the immune system is fortified, we are far less likely to be stricken—or to succumb to common or degenerative health problems, even cancer. Consider the study conducted by a team of researchers at the University of Texas Cancer Center. They exposed bacteria to certain cancer-causing chemicals (carcinogens) together in the accompaniment of a live sprout assortment. They found that the cancer cells were "99 percent inhibited" by the mix of live sprouts.[25] Statistically speaking, this would suggest that live sprouts indeed have the ability to inhibit cancer cells, full stop. Obviously not in every case, but they certainly play a significant role.

At the risk of irritating some medical doctors, please allow me to share this story with you. Doctors don't like anecdotes when it comes to medical research, but this is no fairy tale. My sister-in-law encouraged my father-in-law to go to the raw foods cleansing center in California I was telling you about earlier. He had been diagnosed with prostate cancer. My sister-in-law wanted her dad to incorporate this living foods approach with the conventional medical treatments to combat the prostate cancer. While recently at the center, my father-in-law was approached by two separate robust gentlemen, one in his sixties and the other who claims eighty-four, but those in the know say he is actually eighty-eight. Nonetheless, these men confessed to having contracted prostate cancer seven years ago and twelve years ago respectively. And both claim to be free of the disease today! These men are convinced that the raw foods and sprouts diet cleared them of cancer, as they confided to my father-in-law. They also told him of several other men who are now free of prostate and other cancers since implementing the living foods diet.

This is powerful stuff. And these are not the only interesting success stories. I have seen many cases where people have cleared their warts, blemishes, facial spots, and other benign growths while eating a strict raw foods and sprouts diet. I am not saying that it works for everyone, but it is certainly one key path to perfect health. I am also not suggesting that people with cancer ought to abandon the traditional medical treatments. In fact, to the contrary; I would always request that any cancer patient undergo conventional medical treatment, but perhaps complement it with the living foods approach, subject to the doctor's approval. Such patients must consult their medical doctors or specialists first.

In order to maintain credibility with the medical establishment and present a cogent argument to you, I wish to cite one last recent study. Researchers at the world-renowned Johns Hopkins University School of Medicine discovered in 1997 that certain sprouted vegetables contain far greater doses of anticancer properties than the regular non-sprouted vegetable.[26] They showed, for example, that where broccoli seeds were used to grow broccoli sprouts instead of conventional broccoli, there was a release of thirty to fifty times more anticancer compounds. These anticancer compounds, called *isothiocyanates,* are already known as potent stimulators of natural detoxifying enzymes, and are considered to be the main reason why green vegetables are such powerful anticancer agents. Reporting in the September 1997 issue of the *Proceedings of the National Academy of Sciences,* Dr. J. W. Fahey, Dr. Yueshing Zhang, and Dr. Paul Talalay explained that the sprout extracts of isothiocyanates caused a reduction in the amount, size, and frequency of tumors in experiments on rats exposed to common carcinogens.[27] Evaluating the results, Dr. John W. Erdman, Director of Nutritional Sciences at the University of Illinois commented, "If you look at the epidemiological data, it's so clear that consumption (of sprouts) is related to a lower cancer risk." Dr. Erdman now recommends that everybody eat a small portion of sprouts daily.

Finally, it is interesting to note that the lead researcher of this Johns Hopkins University study, Dr. Paul Talalay, says that he personally now downs a sprig of sprouts each day as his mid-morning snack. I think that speaks volumes. I always tell my own patients to find out (if you can) what your own doctor does personally, or what would the doctor do for his own mother. For example, if a surgeon says "we should operate"—the key question is, would this doctor recommend the same surgery or the same treatment for his own mother, his own child, his wife, or himself?

That also speaks volumes. So when Dr. Talalay, the chief researcher for the Johns Hopkins University study, confides that he personally has started to eat a daily dose of sprouts, we should all take note.

I'll never forget when a friend of mine was a medical intern at a training hospital in Chicago. The supervising doctor recommended a hysterectomy to a patient. But my friend, the medical intern attending the case, said he could never have personally recommended a hysterectomy to his own mother under the same circumstances.

Nonetheless, Dr. Talalay and his colleagues at Johns Hopkins want us to know that when you eat sprouts, you conserve the body's energy, simultaneously enhancing immunity and reducing your risk of cancer. Much of the reason is because sprouts have a high natural concentration of antioxidant nutrients, which combat the effects of free radicals. Free radicals are highly reactive fragments of molecules produced from undesirable oxygen reactions and fat metabolism in our cell membranes. This happens when cells use nutrients and oxygen to make basic energy, and when the body carries out its ordinary metabolic breakdown of organic compounds. It is a normal process, therefore, for our bodies to create these damaging molecules. But our bodies will create even more of these damaging molecules when exposed to chemical pollutants, food additives, radiation, stress, and more. Excess free radicals are often created by poorly digested food, as well, especially rancid or overheated fats and oils, which stress the immune system.

Biochemically, these fragmented molecules are not "electronically" balanced; they are one electron short. In an effort to balance themselves, the unpaired molecule will steal an electron from another pair of nearby balanced molecules. Robbed of its partner molecule, the now electronically unbalanced molecule will in turn steal a partner electron from its neighbor and so on. It is a chain reaction of internal destruction, which, if left unchecked, will cause disease as well as accelerate the aging process.

When free radicals enter our cells, the genetic material of the cell—or DNA—is damaged. Cells also can harden, preventing nutrient uptake; in some cases the cells collapse, their fluid drains away, and you end up with wrinkles and saggy skin, perhaps prematurely. Cell damage will be less if there are plenty of essential nutrients, water, antioxidants, and enzymes available to the body. Just by being alive, undesirable oxygen reactions will destroy our cells. Antioxidants, however, control the actions of oxygen; they prevent or slow down the damage. Antioxidants, like vitamins A, C, and E, are found in abundance in living foods such as sprouts.

The Digestion Connection

Sprouts are excellent for improving and supporting the digestive system because of their extraordinarily high concentration of vitamins, minerals, and live active enzymes. When sprouts are consumed at their optimum growing stage, the nutrients contained within the seeds are already partially digested, and therefore much easier for the body to absorb.

Poor digestion can also result in a buildup of mucus; mucus can then accumulate in the lungs causing shortness of breath, wheezing, asthma, and persistent coughs. Sprouts counteract the effect of mucus-producing foods by reducing moisture and assisting with its removal from the body. Sprouts play a role in the breakdown of fats, proteins, and starches, again enabling easier digestion. If you need to lose weight, eating sprouts is like a virtual panacea.

The Liver Connection

Sprouts are also alkaline, which helps to neutralize acid waste matter, producing cleansing and cooling effects in the body. Therefore, sprouts stimulate the liver energy flow. Most liver imbalances are caused as a result of stagnation. Sprouts assist by stimulating the liver back into normal function. Signs of liver disorder might include nervous tension, depression, frustration, swollen abdomen, bloating, and unexplained lumps and swellings.

ACIDOSIS SELF-EVALUATION

Watch your own acid–alkaline progress as you embark on a sprouts program. Buy Nitrazine paper at a chemist or pharmacy. Apply your urine to the paper, either before eating, or one hour after. The paper will change color to indicate if your system is overly acidic. Once you are regularly eating sprouts, you could perform this acidosis self-evaluation each week, and hopefully, witness your biochemistry improve.

The Clinical Connection

I see many people at my clinic who are suffering from acidosis (tissue toxemia), a condition in which the body is simply too acidic. If you don't eat enough alkaline-forming foods (rich in magnesium, calcium, and potassium), like live sprouts, fresh fruits, vegetables, salads, and millet, you can create an acid stomach. When the body is too acid, it provides a fertile ground for acute and chronic diseases. Kidney, liver, and adrenal disorders, poor diet, obesity, stress, and toxemia can create acidosis. Stress, sugar, animal products, dairy, eggs, and even too many grains such as wheat, might have an acidifying effect on the body. When metabolized, these foods produce large amounts of chlorine and toxins. Symptoms of acidosis can include stomach ulcers, insomnia, headaches, gas, bloating, foul-smelling stools, water retention, arthritis, and other more serious health problems, such as cancer and heart disease.

An acid body means that there is an excess of hydrogen ions, which combine with oxygen to form water. This excess hydrogen depletes the body's oxygen. Simply stated, a shortage of oxygen causes cells to break down and die, creating acidosis. The more acidic the system, the less the biochemical buffers are able to maintain the blood's healthy acid-alkaline balance. A more serious consequence of acidity is that it causes calcium to be mobilized out of your bones through urine; such conditions create a fertile ground for conditions like osteoporosis and bone degeneration. Excess acid may also get deposited in cell tissues, eventually causing arthritis. Live sprouts, especially sprouted millet, are alkalizers; they mop up acid. When I prescribe patients the sprouted millet and sprouted quinoa together, the acid neutralizes: it appears that when these two specific sprouts, millet and quinoa, are ingested together, there is an exceptionally powerful alkalizing action.

HOW TO SPROUT SEEDS AND BEANS

You can easily sprout seeds and beans at home. Try clover, alfalfa seeds, mung beans, fenugreek, and wheat berries, for example.

All you need is a large jam jar (1-quart jars are even better), some seeds or beans, fresh water, and a piece of cheesecloth or muslin.

1. Rinse the seeds well. Place in the jar and cover with a few centimeters of cooled, boiled water. Cover with cheesecloth, or net cloth secured with a rubber band and leave overnight in a warm, dark place.

2. Rinse the seeds next day with fresh water. Drain well or the seeds will rot. Return to the dark. Do this twice a day until seeds start to sprout. Tilt your jar to a 45-degree angle to allow the sprouts to grow up the jar.

3. Then place them on a sunny windowsill for a few hours to give them an energy boost. Eat, or store in an airtight container in the fridge. Sprouts will keep in the fridge for two to three days.

If you want to grow lots of sprouts, purchase a sprouting tray kit from a garden center or health shop. These kits come with easy-to-follow instructions. The extra space provided by the trays will allow your sprouts to grow taller and more abundant. Alternatively, use a kitchen colander or bamboo basket. Baskets should be sterilized by boiling them for approximately three minutes. The openings or holes need to be small so that the seeds do not fall out.

Protect your sprouts with a loose plastic cover. The plastic needs to be thick enough (4 millimeters approximately) so that it stands up erect. You are essentially creating a tent around your basket. It needs to stand erect to allow air to circulate and to retain moisture and temperature. If the plastic covering falls on top of your sprouts, it will damage them. Your cover can stand approximately 25 centimeters high. Elevate your basket a little with a couple of stones or kitchen utensils. This prevents direct contact with the plastic. You need to clean the plastic regularly to avoid mold growth.

The Simple Steps

1. Soak seeds overnight in a jar.

2. Pour seeds into your colander or basket.

3. Rinse evenly.

4. Place basket in plastic tent.

5. Rinse sprouts for thirty seconds, twice daily.

Rinse Note: Tap spray adaptors (flexible spray hoses attached to the sink) much like the showerhead in a shower are ideal for rinsing your sprouts. (A filtering attachment is important to purify the water.) These spray adaptors allow you to water the seeds evenly and is less forceful than the full velocity of water from the regular tap head. You can also use a watering can.

Many seeds are ready within twenty-four hours. Others may take up to seventy-two hours or three to five days. If you leave your sprouts too long, their roots will grow really long and become bitter in taste. Do not keep sprouts past five or six days.

Some sprouts—that is, lentils and mung beans—will be easier on the digestion once the hulls (or shells) are removed. When your lentil sprouts are ready to harvest, put a strainer into a large bowl and pour the lentils into the strainer. Run water over your lentils, squeezing the sprouts to remove the hulls. The hulls on mung beans are tougher to remove; therefore, soaking with warm water a couple of times should do the trick. Other sprouts such as fenugreek or alfalfa simply require rinsing.

Seeds	Soaking Time (hrs)	Sprouting Time (days)	Quantity	Yield
Adzuki	4-5	3-5	1 cup	2-3 cups
Alfalfa	4-6	3-5	3 tbsp	3 cups
Amaranth	4-6	2-3	3 tbsp	3⁄4 cup
Anise	4-6	2	3 tbsp	1 cup
Barley	8-10	3-4	$\frac{1}{2}$ cup	1 cup
Most beans	8-10	3-5	1 cup	3-4 cups
Buckwheat	4-6	2-3	1 cup	2-3 cups
Cabbage	4-6	2-3	1 tbsp	$1\frac{1}{2}$ cups
Chia	4-6	1-4	1 tbsp	$1\frac{1}{2}$ cups
Chickpeas (garbanzo)	10-12	3	1 cup	3 cups
Clover	4-6	3-5	1 tbsp	$2\frac{1}{2}$ cups
Corn	8-10	2-3	1 cup	2 cups
Fenugreek (spicy)	4-6	3-5	4 tbsp	1 cup
Flax	5-7	4	1 tbsp	1 cup
Green peas	10-12	3	1 cup	2 cups
Lentils	6-8	3	1 cup	3-4 cups

Seeds	Soaking Time (hrs)	Sprouting Time (days)	Quantity	Yield
Millet	6-8	3-4	1 cup	1$\frac{1}{2}$ cups
Mung beans	8-10	3-5	1 cup	3-4 cups
Mustard	4-6	3-4	1 tbsp	1 cup
Most nuts	8-12	3-5	1 cup	1$\frac{1}{2}$ cups
Oats	8-10	3-4	1 cup	2 cups
Onion	4-6	2-3	1 tbsp	1 cup
Pumpkin seeds	6-8	3	1 cup	1$\frac{1}{2}$ cups
Quinoa	4-6	2-3	1 cup	2$\frac{1}{2}$ cups
Radish (spicy)	4-6	2-6	1 tbsp	1 cup
Rice	8-10	3-4	1 cup	1$\frac{1}{2}$ cups
Rye	8-10	3-4	1 cup	2$\frac{1}{2}$ cups
Sesame seeds	4-6	3	1 cup	1$\frac{1}{2}$ cups
Soybeans	10-12	4-6	1 cup	2$\frac{1}{2}$ cups
Sunflower seeds	6-8	1-3	1 cup	1$\frac{1}{2}$ cups
Watercress	4-6	2-3	1 tbsp	1$\frac{1}{2}$ cups
Wheat	10-12	2-4	1 cup	2$\frac{1}{2}$ cups

Easiest to Sprout	Hard to Sprout
Adzuki	Barley
Alfalfa	Chia
Clover	Chickpeas
Fenugreek (spicy)	(garbanzo)
Green/red peas	Flax
Lentils	Millet
Mung beans	Quinoa
Radish (spicy)	Rice
Rye	Soybean
Wheat	Hulled sunflower

Voilà! You can become a sprout chef after all!

3.

MILLET:
Digestion Dynamo

NUTRITIONALLY:
high in iron, magnesium, potassium, silicon, the B vitamins and vitamin E.

PHYSIOLOGICALLY:
supports the digestive organs, especially the stomach and spleen (your energy battery).

BENEFITS:
more energy. Assists digestion, improving nutrient uptake. Removes unwanted excess acid and helps to inhibit growth of fungus and nasty yeasts.

I have learned through the years that most people are creatures of habit, eating roughly the same things every day. "I always have a baked potato at lunch time," one patient boasts. I grew up on meat and potatoes in the highlands of Scotland, so I can completely relate to this.

British people taught the Western world to love potatoes so much that in many cases they're eaten with nearly every meal. By now, it must be in our genes! Potato genes! I can remember years ago, when I was embarking on life-changing food plans, not feeling happy if I could not have potatoes with my meal. I felt unsatisfied, empty, almost as if I had not eaten. I would be totally discontented with the meal. There is nothing wrong with potatoes in moderation, but day in day out, twice daily, year in year out, may not be such a good idea. Ultimately, too many potatoes in your diet can have an unhealthy acidifying effect on the body.[28]

I think of potatoes as a "wet" food. In other words, too many potatoes provide our bodies with an environment for mucus production. A massive amount of the population eats potatoes and also suffers from mucus and fungal conditions. I am not saying that potatoes are the cause of all mucus and fungal conditions, but when eaten in abundance and continuously, they in fact can create some problems. If you eat the same food every single day, it can almost become toxic to the body. That's why I always recommend that you rotate foods for balance: don't eat the same foods every day; give your body a rest.

Here is where millet comes in. Since millet can be made to taste and look similar to mashed potatoes, it makes for an excellent alternative to potatoes. And finally, because millet is an antifungal, antimucus agent, plus digestive aid, it becomes even more attractive. To learn how to prepare my Millet Mashed Potatoes recipe (instead of mashed potatoes), see page 40. Millet is more commonly eaten as a cooked grain, but it can be sprouted to gain even more nutritional benefits. It has been used as a bird food in the West for many years, yet the Chinese have been eating sprouted millet for centuries calling it the "queen of grains."

NUTRITIONAL ELEMENTS

Sprouted millet provides an excellent source of iron, the B vitamins, and fiber. It delivers low-calorie protein and also contains significant amounts of silicon, niacin, thiamine, riboflavin, magnesium, potassium, and a moderate amount of vitamin E. As with most sprouted seeds and grains, millet is a rich source of digestive enzymes. Millet is also gluten-free, and therefore can be consumed freely by those suffering from intolerance to wheat and other allergenic foods.

The Digestive Aid

Including millet, either sprouted or in grain form, in your diet is an excellent way of supporting your digestive organs: the stomach, spleen, and pancreas. Your stomach needs the strength to receive and digest food; *your spleen must extract the lipids (fats) from that food and convert them into energy fuel for the body.* Your pancreas needs to release digestive enzymes into your system to help break down proteins, fats, and carbohydrates.

Millet contains the nutritional compounds and food energies that have a stabilizing effect on the stomach, spleen, and pancreas, enabling them to perform their functions better. Biochemical molecules restore a flow of energy and balance between these three interconnected organs so critical to optimum digestion.

When I look at a cross-section of my patient portfolio, it is safe to say that more than 80 percent of those who first came to consult with me were complaining of symptoms linked to gastrointestinal distress. Through biochemical evaluation and stool analysis, it is usually clear to me that one or more of the key organs of digestion are compromised and weakened in their digestive functions. At my practice, I use millet in various forms as part of a dietary plan for patients in need of improved digestion. Chronic indigestion, gas, bloating, burping, belching, stomach ulcers, bad breath (usually a sign of poor digestion and bacteria buildup), and acidosis all respond well to the inclusion of this remarkable food.

Case Study: Mr. Farthington, Diabetic

Mr. Farthington, now sings my praises (he really deserves the credit though) for insisting that he include millet, twice weekly, in his diet. Mr. Farthington was an avid potato eater, up to three times daily, not including his daily bag of potato chips. Millet is a must for diabetics, as it clears stomach heat (acidosis), a common side effect of the condition, and cools down the overactive stomach compounds responsible for indigestion. Millet nourishes the digestive organs with its positive effect on the pancreas, the enzyme-producing organ. The pancreas is also better able to produce hormones to regulate blood sugar levels. Balanced blood sugar levels are critical for the diabetic. Mr. Farthington is now using millet in soups, vegetable dishes, and casseroles, and as a cereal. Check out my millet recipes to learn how you, too, can benefit.

Tongues and Millet

Please allow me to share my millet story with you about a fifty-one-year-old patient named Edna, who was recovering from a surgical operation. She had suffered substantial blood loss, transfusions, and of course disrupted digestion. Feeling weak, she was desperate for more energy. When Edna came to my clinic, she was amazed when I ordered her to stick out her tongue. After tongue analysis, my suspicions were confirmed. Edna was suffering from a severe spleen deficiency and weakened stomach.

Tongue analysis is just one diagnostic tool I use in my practice to evaluate a patient. It's like a window to your insides, with each area of the tongue correlating to a different organ. I also use an array of biochemical tests utilizing urine, stool, sweat, and blood. Such biochemical tests tend to almost always confirm my initial tongue analysis.

Edna had deep scalloped edges around the sides of her tongue, similar to teeth marks. This is a give-away for a sluggish spleen. And she had a midline tongue crack, indicating a weak digestion. Edna gladly embarked on my nutritional recommendations to strengthen her digestive organs. Warm millet, as well as some sprouted millet, became part of her regimen. She reported back to me almost immediately after incorporating warm cooked millet into her diet. She could feel the difference in her energy levels; Edna credited the millet with her health improvement. I am pleased to report that after a year on my program, Edna no longer suffers from spleen weakness.

HEALTH BENEFITS

Sprouted millet can be used successfully to counteract acidity within the digestive tract because of its alkalinity factor. If you do not eat enough alkaline-forming foods, such as sprouts and fresh fruit and vegetables, you can create an acid environment in the stomach. This leads to a lack of oxygen, causing the cells to break down and die. Because of this alkalinity factor, sprouted millet neutralizes acid in the body. Acidity, when advanced, causes calcium to be leached out of the bones, and excreted through the urine. Excess acid can ultimately degrade the cell tissues, leading to arthritis and even gout.

Too much acid, a common problem referred to as acidosis, can trigger stomach ulcers, heartburn, gas, bloating, foul-smelling stools, bad breath and body odor, poor mental and physical performance, general aches and pains, and unexplained anger. Acidosis is a common cause of yeast-related conditions such as *Candida albicans*. As a source of antifungal compounds, millet can help to inhibit the growth of yeast, *Candida albi-cans,* and other pathogenic conditions. In summary, sprouted millet helps to remove acid from the system, rendering the body more alkaline and less prone to acidic related ailments.

In its sprouted form, millet helps to strengthen and support the digestive system by introducing valuable enzymes. Consequently, it may alleviate dryness, chapped lips, dry skin, constipation, and unproductive coughs.

From a nutritional standpoint, millet is especially rich in both potassium and magnesium. Potassium counteracts excess salt consumption, whether by the addition of salt on food, or the hidden salt found in many processed foods. The magnesium stimulates calcium production, thereby strengthening calcium bone density in the quest to prevent such problems as arthritis or osteoporosis. Millet's rich silicon content helps to rebuild connective tissue, also vital to the arterial and skeletal system.

From a physiological approach, millet also detoxifies and cools the liver, and harmonizes and nurtures the kidneys. Millet supports the spleen, pancreas, and stomach. If these organs become deficient, the kidneys will be required to work harder, thus establishing a chain reaction domino effect. Signs of kidney overload are often extreme exhaustion, agitation, irritation, nervousness, insecurity, fear, running from one problem to another, and a sense of being not "rooted."

Clinical Note

In my clinical practice, I have used millet to aid in the prevention of miscarriage and morning sickness in pregnant women, and I recommend it to reduce stomach problems such as diarrhea and indigestion. I wish to share a particular case of a patient, Eleanor, who overcame severe spleen weakness with the help of sprouted millet. She had a history of miscarriages, a sign in itself of a sluggish spleen. After finally giving birth to her only child, she was consistently exhausted, bloated, and suffered heartburn, flatulence, and yeast overgrowth. Through biochemical testing, I discovered low levels of the minerals magnesium, zinc, chromium, and manganese. She was practically devoid of any hydrochloric acid enzymes and other digestive juices in the stomach (common for spleen weakness patients).

She embarked upon my program, including a rotation of sprouted millet or cooked millet as a side dish with at least one meal each day for thirty days. I then started her on a sprouted millet powder along with certain botanicals specifically beneficial for the spleen: including a rotation of astragalus, ginseng, pau d'arco, and wild blue-green algae. She was also taking vitamin E and supplementary digestive enzymes.

Within sixty days Eleanor reported "amazing energy, no more gas, bloating, or indigestion." After about ninety days on my program, the candida yeast overgrowth subsided. And one major bonus: Eleanor no longer had hemorrhoids, a problem she had endured for years (hemorrhoids, in fact, are another classic sign of a weak spleen and congested liver). The introduction of millet for this patient was exceedingly efficacious.

Millet, sprouted and in grain form, is easy to digest and is free from gluten, a common allergen. More specifically, millet is an antifungal agent, high in iron, magnesium, and silicon, which builds cell tissue for healthy bones, hair, skin and nails.

USING MILLET

Eat millet grain two to three times weekly if you can. It is a marvelous addition to our modern lifestyles. Use it in soups, salads, stews, and by itself. You'll be glad you did.

Millet is simple to make:

BASIC MILLET

3 cups water

1 cup millet

herbal seasoning or sea salt to taste

Bring water and millet to a boil.

Simmer for 25 minutes.

The millet should absorb the liquid and be soft.

Season to taste.

MILLET-MASHED POTATOES

1 onion, chopped fresh

1 cauliflower, cut into small pieces (approx 2 cups)

2 cups millet

7 cups water

¼ cup chopped fresh parsley

sea salt to taste

Place the onion, cauliflower, and millet in layers in a saucepan. Add the water, cover, and bring to a boil.

Reduce the heat and simmer for 25 minutes. Millet should absorb liquid and be soft. Drain off excess water before mashing. Mash or purée in a food processor. Add a little water if necessary. Usually, I blend only half of the mixture. I mix this into the unblended ingredients for a more chewy consistency.

Garnish with raw parsley. Season with sea salt to taste.

You'll think you're eating potatoes! Yet, your body will be enjoying a welcome change.

Serve the Millet Mashed Potatoes with Onion Gravy.

ONION GRAVY

2 large onions, sliced

1 teaspoon oil

2 cups spring water

2 teaspoons wheat-free tamari sauce or soy sauce

1½ tablespoons kudzu (plant used as a thickener—
helps strengthen digestive tract; comes in powder form)

sea salt to taste

Place thinly sliced onions in a pan with warm oil. Do not overheat. Cook at a low temperature, browning the onions. Add 2 cups of water; simmer for 10 minutes.

Mix together tamari and kudzu in cold water. Kudzu should dissolve.

Add mixture to simmering onions. Stir until liquid becomes clear and thicker.

Add sea salt for seasoning.

Pour over Millet Mashed Potatoes.

Absolutely delicious!

You can use a vegetable bouillon cube in place of the soy sauce or tamari sauce. Kudzu and tamari can be purchased in health food stores. Use your own gravy or thickener if you prefer.

Q: WHO MAY BENEFIT FROM MILLET?
A: EVERYONE

Millet will support your digestive organs. Its nutritional compounds and food energies have a stabilizing effect on your stomach and digestive function. Millet compounds will help relieve the body of acid toxins.

Also, utilizing millet in your diet will give your body a rest from the more common grains, such as wheat.

4.

QUINOA:
The Most Powerful Protein

NUTRITIONALLY:
more usable protein than meat, containing all the essential amino
acids: a rich source of minerals including more usable calcium than
milk.

PHYSIOLOGICALLY:
supports the kidneys.

BENEFITS:
enhances bones and sexual prowess (good sex depends on well-
functioning kidneys!)

Growing up in Scotland, I know there's not a mother "worth her salt" who
will send her "wee bairn" to school in the winter without a hot bowl of
(oat) porridge. "It'll stick tae yer ribs," my mum used to say. That sounded
pretty scary, but Mum actually had a good point. Biochemically speaking,
warm oatmeal will keep your insides cozy, and therefore help you battle
through those cold, damp mornings (provided that the oatmeal is not
laden with sugar and swimming in cow's milk!). But you're bound to get fed
up with oatmeal every day. I did. After thousands of bowls of sticky oatmeal, I then couldn't face it for years! I once calculated that from the age
of three until seventeen years old (when I left home to attend Edinburgh
University) I had insisted on eating in excess of 17,600 bowls of oatmeal.

So, what's an alternative? Enter quinoa. Make your loved ones a quinoa
oatmeal instead. It will be a welcome change for oatmeal addicts. Serious-

ly though, quinoa will do for your kidneys what Scottish oatmeal is supposed to do for your ribs! It will warm them up, and give you a feeling of satisfaction. And on those chilly mornings, you'll feel warm all over after a bowl of quinoa oatmeal. I'm not suggesting that you eat 17,600 bowls of quinoa during a major period of your life, but feel free to use it as a viable alternative some of the time. When I make this suggestion to parents, the most common retort is always, "my kids won't like it." That's where they are wrong. Let the kids try it. Give it a go yourself. Mix it with another grain that you are more familiar with, if it makes you happier about trying it.

My five-year-old child actually loves quinoa! She herself requests it, more so in the winter because she feels so good after eating it. Quinoa strengthens the kidneys. The kidney strength of your child influences growth, development, and ability to learn. Although our basic constitutional kidney strength is inherited from our parents, we can build on that inherited constitution and strengthen the kidneys by eating the right foods, like quinoa. It's that simple.

In Eastern medical philosophy, strong kidneys are the foundation and root of all bodily functions. For example, good sex, and the ability to reproduce, will depend on reasonable kidney function. Good hearing, healthy breathing, the condition of your hair, lack of urinary problems, bone marrow production, brain function, the will to succeed in life, strong teeth and bones, all depend on healthy functioning kidneys. They are your gateway to vitality in life. You need to think of your kidneys as your "lot in life," your starting point, your constitutional strength. They are a bit like having a bank account. You can either gain interest by strengthening them, or go into overdraft by weakening them. So if you constantly make excessive demands on your body by eating the wrong foods, you will weaken your most fundamental right at having a healthy life. You will go into kidney debt. The kidneys are your source of "heat" for your body, your solid rock as well. If you feel cold a lot and/or have dark circles under your eyes, suffer anxiety, mental fatigue, back pain, crave salty foods, are overly emotional, suffer hair or bone problems, or have undigested food in your stools, then you definitely must start eating quinoa to strengthen the kidneys.

Quinoa is commonly referred to as a cereal grain, but technically it is really the botanical fruit of an herb plant. It was a staple of the ancient Incas, who called it the "mother grain," and it is still an important food in Central and South America today. Quinoa (pronounced *keen-wah*) "grains" are small, yellow, flat spheres, approximately 1.5 to 2 mm in diameter. When cooked, the seed-like germ coils into a small "tail" that lends a pleasant crunch. It is cooked in a similar way to rice, but takes about half the time, and expands to four times its original volume.

Its flavor is delicate, almost bland, and is often compared to that of couscous. Because some of the bitter saponin covering on quinoa can still be present, even though most is washed before being sold, you should thoroughly rinse the dry "grain" until the water runs clear. Quinoa is a very versatile food and can be served in many ways, including as a hot cereal, pudding, or a cold grain in salads, or added to soups and stews. It can also be sprouted, which is not only delicious but enhances the nutritional value.

NUTRITIONAL ELEMENTS

The nutritional content of sprouted quinoa is impressive. It is extremely high in protein and low in fat, and has virtually no cholesterol. In its sprouted form, quinoa contains vitamins A, B_6, B_{12}, C, D, E, and K, biotin, folic acid, niacin, pantothenic acid, riboflavin, and thiamine. It is a rich source of the minerals iron and calcium with traces of chromium, copper, fluoride, iodine, magnesium, manganese, molybdenum, phosphorus, potassium, selenium, and zinc. And it contains all nine of the essential amino acids. Thus, sprouted quinoa is a more efficient and more digestible form of protein than meat.

Although the protein level of quinoa compares to, or even surpasses, many meats, this form of vegetable protein does not lead to cholesterol or hardening of the arteries. In fact, the opposite is true. Sprouted quinoa is cleansing to the heart and arterial system. It reduces the amount of fat in the blood and it actually prevents arterial plaque, thereby reducing the risk of a stroke or heart attack. Therefore, regularly eating quinoa, especially sprouted quinoa, decreases the risk of heart problems. Regularly eating red meat, on the other hand, dramatically increases the risk of heart disease.

Vital for Vegetarians

Quinoa can be a very important addition to a vegetarian diet, since plants frequently have amino acid deficiencies. Wheat, corn, and rice are deficient in the amino acid lysine for example. Beans, lentils, and other legumes are deficient in the amino acid cysteine. Amino acids are the building blocks for proteins. The nine essential amino acids cannot be produced by the body in sufficient quantity for normal bodily functions. Therefore, complete protein can only be created by the food we eat. Without all the essential amino acids, the body cannot make complete protein. Amino acid deficiency may result in reduced growth, anemia, muscular degeneration, emaciation, or worse.

This may explain why many of the vegetarians who initially arrive at my clinic are so weak and so nutritionally deficient, according to biochemical tests. By regularly eating the sprouted quinoa, these vegetarians or vegans begin to shift their nutritional profiles. For the first time, they are ingesting correct amounts of protein and other nutrients. As a result, their energy levels, sexual desires, and quality of the hair, skin, and nails dramatically improve within relatively short periods of time.

Quinoa also contains more calcium than milk and therefore helps to support the skeletal system, bone, and cartilage. Thus, quinoa can serve as a protector against arthritis, bone degeneration, calcium malabsorption, and other related disorders.

Love Your Liver

From the physiological perspective, sprouted quinoa can also be particularly useful in strengthening and revitalizing another critical organ, the liver. Because quinoa is a warming food, it can help to reduce damp or mucus in the liver. The liver is the largest and perhaps most important organ, as it performs some 600 different functions. The liver is the major detoxifier for the body—responsible for ridding it of pollutants, chemicals, and other foreign agents. Finally, the flow of energy through the body is a most important job of the liver. If this organ is compromised, there is no doubt that you will be absolutely exhausted. But if we revitalize and restore the liver, you will definitely feel the difference.

Physical signs of a stagnant liver may include nervous system disorders, allergies, lumps, swelling, chronic indigestion, menstrual problems, stress, neck and back tension, impure blood, skin disorders, exhaustion especially in the morning, tendon problems, and a wiry, tight radial pulse.

More subtle emotional signs of a stagnant liver can include anger, frustration, resentment, impatience, edginess, depression, moodiness, impulsiveness, mental rigidity, emotional attachments, poor judgment, difficulty making decisions, and negativity. If you suffer from any of these physical or emotional symptoms, then you may have a sluggish liver. Therefore, the inclusion of quinoa in the diet can be particularly beneficial in preventing organ stagnation and ultimately in rejuvenating the liver and kidneys.

USING QUINOA

Use quinoa grain two to three times weekly; more in the winter, especially if you feel cold.

QUINOA PORRIDGE

2 cups water

1 cup quinoa

sea salt to taste

Boil water.

Add quinoa to water, season with sea salt and cover and simmer for approximately 20 minutes. Quinoa should absorb the water and have a fluffy texture. It is incredibly filling and warming to the body. There's a saying, "go to work on an egg." I think it is much better to go to work on Quinoa Porridge.

For a Change

Sometimes, I will put a strip of seaweed into my Quinoa Porridge. This is just to provide a little variety and additional mineral boost. The sea vegetable wakame is my choice to partner with quinoa. It only requires 10 minutes soaking time and has a delicate flavor.

QUINOA SALAD

1 cup quinoa

1 vegetable bouillon cube

sea salt, pinch

salad leaves

few cherry tomatoes

2 celery stalks, diced

1 red onion, thinly sliced

2 red peppers, cut in square cubes

1 carrot, diced

fresh herb of your choice, to garnish

juice of lemon

Rinse quinoa and drain off excess water.

Prepare Quinoa Porridge, adding the vegetable bouillon to the 2 cups water in the recipe.

Bring water to a boil and simmer 20 minutes.

Mix together salad ingredients and garnish with the herb of your choice. My favorites include parsley or dill.

Squeeze lemon juice all over salad.

Serve warm quinoa in the middle of your crispy salad. Sometimes, I even add a few slices of avocado.

Alternatively

Add some pasta sauce for flavor.

Q: WHO MAY BENEFIT FROM QUINOA?
A: EVERYONE (ESPECIALLY THOSE LIVING IN COLD, DAMP CLIMATES)

Quinoa strengthens our kidneys, the root of all of our bodily functions. Our kidneys run the risk of being depleted when we live in cold, damp climates.

Too much stress, little sleep, "burning the candle at both ends," poor food choices also weaken kidney function.

A biweekly infusion of quinoa can help to keep our kidney function vital.

5.

ALFALFA:
The Terrific Tonic

NUTRITIONALLY:

highest in natural digestive enzymes and bioflavonoids, as well as most vitamins, minerals, amino acids, and four times more vitamin C than most citrus fruit.

PHYSIOLOGICALLY:

nourishes your blood and guts. Tonifies intestines and digestive energies.

BENEFITS:

regulates digestive disorders, heartburn, gas, bloating, malabsorption. Beneficial in the breakdown of fat, cellulose, starch.

The name of this powerful plant is derived from the Arabic *al-fal-fa,* "father of all foods," and with very good reason. Alfalfa contains all the known vitamins and minerals necessary for life. And the chlorophyll that is extracted from it has a balance of organic, molecular, and mineral constituents almost identical to human hemoglobin.

With clover-like leaves and purplish flowers, alfalfa is indigenous to Western Asia and the eastern Mediterranean. The Spanish took alfalfa seeds with them to South America in the early 1550s, and it was introduced to the United States by European immigrants in 1736. It is now grown extensively for use as an herbal supplement and general nutritive tonic. A member of the pea and bean family, alfalfa has an extensive root system that can reach depths of over 100 feet, and instances have been recorded of these roots touching miners' helmets! Such a powerfully rooted plant can in turn benefit the root or foundation of the human body. Our "roots" are often identified physiologically as the kidneys and intestines.[29] When these "root" organs are efficiently nourished and working optimally, we ought to experience a raised level of well-being and strength. Such long roots give this plant unsurpassed access to minerals and compounds at the deepest level in the soil.

SUPERNUTRIENTS

I consider alfalfa to be a superfood because of the vast array of nutrients it contains. These include eight digestive enzymes, phytoestrogens (plant-based hormones), bioflavonoids (antioxidant, anti-inflammatory, oxygen-based compounds that enhance strength of veins, blood vessels, and capillaries), saponins (a restorative containing mineral salts), flavone (aids fragile capillaries), glycosides (antitumoral compounds), alkaloids (anti-infective, anti-inflammatory plant compounds to help form proteins), amino acids, organic acids, minerals and certain trace minerals (including calcium, magnesium, phosphorus, iron, and potassium), chlorophyll, folic acid, niacin, and vitamins A, B—especially B_{12}—C, D, E, and K! It can be used to reduce inflammation in the lungs, making it beneficial for those with asthma, pneumonia, and bronchitis. It has four times the amount of vitamin C of citrus fruit, and its calcium content is easily absorbed and assimilated by the body.[30] Alfalfa contains more than forty different bioflavonoids.

The Many Benefits

Alfalfa acts as a natural deodorizer and infection-fighter, thanks to the high content of chlorophyll and vitamin A. The leaves contain a large percentage of beta-carotene, which encourages a healthy immune system. Alfalfa helps a wide range of conditions; it is most commonly used for detoxifying and enriching the liver, strengthening and purifying the blood, and aiding digestion, and as a general tonic and boost to the immune system.

As a cleansing agent, it neutralizes acids and toxins. Its high fiber content has the ability to absorb and carry intestinal waste from the body, by softening the stools and improving the contracting action of the colon. It can also be useful in relieving water retention—thereby allowing the body to rid itself of further toxins and excess fluid. With its high vitamin K content, alfalfa can be used to encourage healthy blood flow. It strengthens the blood vessels and capillaries, thus preventing spontaneous bleeding. Studies also indicate that alfalfa may prevent high cholesterol and reduce the buildup of fatty deposits in the arteries.[31] Jack Ritchason also cites a "vitamin U" factor, whereby alfalfa has been shown to prevent ulcers in test animals.[32]

Clinically

In my clinical practice, I use alfalfa leaf to nourish the blood and improve digestion. As a digestive aid, with its eight enzymes, alfalfa leaf helps to assimilate protein, fats, and carbohydrates; this ensures that we absorb the maximum amount of nutrients from the foods we eat. In his book *The Energetics of Western Herbs,* Peter Holmes said that taking the herb alfalfa prior to eating can support gastrointestinal function as it facilitates the release of gastric compounds to aid food digestion. Alfalfa can also aid nutrient uptake if taken at the end of a meal.[33] The end result is the reduction or elimination of heartburn, gas, bloating, indigestion, malabsorption, and other gastric maladies. Clinically as well as personally, I have found alfalfa particularly useful for nursing mothers to improve the quality and quantity of breast milk. Alfalfa leaf can have a regulating effect on estrogen levels and can safely be taken throughout pregnancy; the parts of the plant responsible for this effect are called isoflavones.[34] I have successfully used alfalfa to assist such conditions as arthritis, asthma, bad breath and body odor, fungal and yeast infections, diabetes, fever, and edema. It has also been used as a preventative against tumors, possibly fighting cancer, tooth decay (it contains natural fluoride), and osteoporosis.[35]

Case Study: Mr. Sahid, 28, Engineer

Alfalfa (tablets and tea form) was a major focus in Mr. Sahid's nutritional regimen after a serious back operation. He told me that his recovery time was much faster than in a previous operation where he'd remained weakened for months. This time, he regained his strength within a short period and left the hospital earlier than expected.

Case Study: Mrs. Liebner, 38, Mother

Many of my postpartum ladies swear by alfalfa as part of the recovery process after childbirth. Mrs. Liebner claimed that only six weeks after the birth of her third child, she felt her vitality had returned. "It's my lifesaver," (referring to alfalfa), she confessed. Prior to coming to my clinic, she had experienced two difficult postpartum periods with her other children, as well as problems shifting the excess weight. This time, it was so different. "The third time was lucky," she laughed, "but only due to the nutritional support and the restorative abilities of alfalfa."

I congratulated her on her new arrival and urged her to continue the regimen. I asked if there was anything else she needed. "I want four," she quietly whispered. "Four what?" I inquired. "Four children. If I can feel this good, there's no reason why I can't have another. I love being a mum!" I was lost for words, something I'm not usually known for!

USING ALFALFA

You can get alfalfa leaf in tablet, powder, tincture, and tea form. Buy it at your local health food shop. It is best to follow dosage suggestions on the label. However, general suggestions might be:

- Drink 2 cups of alfalfa tea every other day.
- Two 2,000–4,000 mg capsules three times daily
- You can grow your own alfalfa sprouts (see page 30).
- Alfalfa sprouts are high in vitamins, minerals, and amino acids.

Dr. Ben A. Bradley, an American physician who specialized in herbal medicine, wrote in 1915, "I find in alfalfa, after years of clinical tests in my practice and on myself, a superlative restorative tonic. Alfalfa rejuvenates the whole system by increasing the strength, vigor and vitality of the patient."[36] I couldn't have put it better, nearly ninety years later.

Alfalfa leaf nourishes the deepest level of our being, namely the kidneys and intestine function (our guts), thus helping to clear the body of toxins. Tonifying the intestines, alfalfa thus nourishes our blood with important nutrients and is good for combating fatigue, anemia, malabsorption, and heartburn. Alfalfa contains eight live enzymes to break down fat, cellulose, and starch.

ALFALFA QUESTIONNAIRE

If you answer "yes" to one or more of the following questions, you may benefit from alfalfa.

❑ Do you eat processed foods, fast foods, microwaved foods, "boil in the bag" type foods three or more times a week?

❑ Do you suffer from malabsorption?

❑ Look at your tongue: any lines, cracks, or teeth marks?

❑ Do you suffer from heartburn?

❑ Do you experience gas or flatulence?

❑ Are you bloated after eating?

❑ Are you a burper? (that's without beer or wine please!)

❑ Do you have visible capillaries (thread veins) on your nose and cheeks?

❑ Do you suffer from easy bruising?

❑ Have you ever been anemic?

❑ Do you have a pale complexion?

❑ Do you feel weak/vulnerable?

❑ Are you recovering from an operation or have you just given birth?

❑ Is your hair condition poor (dry, brittle)?

❑ Is your stamina low?

❑ Are you tired a lot?

❑ Do you have weight problems?

❑ Is your resistance to infections low?

❑ Have you tested positive for vitamin K deficiency or poor calcium and protein uptake?

❑ Have you experienced repeated miscarriages?

❑ Is your vision poor?

❑ Do you have a history of heart disease?

❑ Do you suffer from nosebleeds?

If you exhibit one to three of the above symptoms, try alfalfa every other day for three to six months.

If you exhibit six to nine of the above symptoms, try alfalfa daily for three to six months.

If you exhibit ten or more symptoms, increase alfalfa dosage as directed on the bottle.

Take for approximately six to nine months on a daily basis.

You also need to add more superfoods into your diet.

6.

ALOE VERA:
Healer and Strengthener

NUTRITIONALLY:
especially rich in plant sterols, amino acids and polysaccharides.

PHYSIOLOGICALLY:
strengthening to all organs and cell tissue. Loves your liver.

BENEFITS:
repairs damaged tissue, reduces inflammation, assists digestion, and
promotes free flow of energy through all meridians.

About a decade ago, when my husband (boyfriend at the time) was going
through major job stress, he collapsed on the beach in pain one summer.
It was bound to happen; it seemed only to be a question of when. He had
been suffering with severe stomach pains, bowel blockages, and constipation, and was probably developing an ulcer until it all caught up with him
in a massive attack. Here was my 6'2", young, vital man flat on the floor,
unable to walk, with shortness of breath, due to the pain. When the doctor (who also happened to be a surgeon) arrived, he suggested that "we
open him up and see what's going on." "What do you mean, 'open him
up'?" I tersely queried. "You know, an operation, exploratory-type," the
surgeon responded. "You mean surgery?" I gasped. "Yes, I think next
Tuesday would be fine," he confirmed.

As my future husband lay there in disbelief, he started to hyperventi-
late, if he wasn't already doing so. Next Tuesday at the hospital never
arrived, only because my man is terrified by white institutional buildings.
The following day, instead, he started to drink $\frac{1}{4}$ cup of aloe vera juice in

¾ cup of apple juice three times each day—only out of desperation. A few days later, he began a course of colonic hydrotherapy treatments, also out of desperation. And the rest was history, as they say. Within three weeks, he was like a new man, and he has never looked back—touch wood.

THE MAIN CONSTITUENTS

Aloe vera is a powerful medicinal plant belonging to the lily family. It has a cactus-like appearance, with thick thorn-edged leaves, which vary in color from gray to bright green. It grows in warm, dry regions: Africa, Asia, South and Central America, Southern Europe, the Caribbean, and other tropical and semitropical areas.

Aloe is called *kumari* in Sanskrit, which means "goddess." It is used by East Indian women to maintain beauty and counteract symptoms of aging. Ayurvedic medicine considers aloe to be estrogenic. This accounts for its vitalizing and tonifying properties for women.

Aloe vera has two main constituents:

1. the gel, which is found inside the leaves;

2. the exudate, which is derived from the juice, obtained from cells beneath the tough outer skin.

Because the exudate contains active substances that have a strong laxative effect, most of this is removed in the extraction process. However, the traces that remain are believed to contribute to the overall effectiveness of aloe vera, aiding the stomach function, intestines, and liver.

The gel part of the aloe vera plant contains many active constituents: these include eighteen amino acids, organic acids, vitamins, minerals, mineral salts, plant hormones and sterols (plant steroids), bradykininase (an enzyme), salicylates (aromatic acids), and polysaccharides (complex sugars). Although some of the nutrients are not strong enough to produce a therapeutic action on their own, the joint "synergistic" effect of all the ingredients together contributes to the efficiency exhibited by aloe vera.

Aloe vera works by initiating four prime activities within the body:

1. anti-inflammatory,

2. antibacterial,

3. immune stimulating,

4. general tissue repair.

Clinically, I often incorporate aloe vera into nutrition programs to help combat yeast-related disorders. Several studies have demonstrated aloe's activity against many common bacteria and fungi.[37] In high concentrations, aloe was found to be effective against much gut-altering pathogens such as *Candida albicans,* citrobacter, klihiella, prendomonas, and more.[38] Naturally occurring caprylic acid, a potent antifungal, has also been found in aloe.[39] When I conduct further analysis on "yeasty" patients, it is not unusual to find one or more negative pathogens, which can cause havoc in the gastrointestinal tract. These gastrointestinal imbalances severely alter the body's natural ecosystem of good bacteria. All kinds of bowel disorders and digestive disturbances can result. Aloe vera can act as a catalyst in the elimination of negative pathogens and microbes.[40]

CLINICAL FINDINGS

At the McKeith Clinic, we routinely conduct biochemical stool analysis of those patients with symptoms of gastrointestinal distress. In many cases, this evaluation of digestion, absorption, intestinal function, and internal environment reveal malabsorption of food and gross imbalances of friendly bacteria. Negative pathogens upset the delicate gut environment, resulting in a state of severely altered bacterial flora—the bad bacteria swamping the good. Patients do not always realize the potential health damage when living with the detrimental effects of a toxic intestinal/ bowel system. These toxins build up over the years and can become the source of many problems. I have found aloe vera to be helpful in the removal and regulation of microbial toxins and intestinal toxicosis.

Trials conducted on the positive use of aloe vera on the gastrointestinal tract seem to support my clinical findings. Trials were conducted by Dr. Jeffrey Bland using aloe vera to determine its effect on gastrointestinal function, stool, and urinary indican. (Urinary indican is an indicator of the degree to which dietary protein is malabsorbed or intestinal bacteria is putrefying.) After one full week of drinking 6 ounces of aloe vera juice three times daily, indican levels of participants decreased.

This result suggests that the aloe vera could improve digestion and assimilation of nutrients, and reduce bacterial putrefaction. In addition, Dr. Bland's trials indicated that the stool was bulkier (healthier), gut flora normalized, and yeast levels lowered.[41] Bowel flora acidophilus products containing live bacteria were not used in this study. The aloe was creating more favorable conditions in which good bacteria would flourish without the use of supplement pills. This living food, aloe, allowed the body to develop its own sources of healthy bacteria naturally, which is what the body should be doing naturally. Once again, the study proved that live foods are the most efficacious medicines.

According to Dr. Bland's study, aloe increased the rate of peristalsis, the wavelike motion that moves waste. This resulted in a faster movement of food passing through the gut. Muscular tone of the intestinal walls had obviously been strengthened. It is no wonder, therefore, that in my practice I should see positive results when using aloe as a core part of programs for such inflammatory gastrointestinal troubles as colitis, diverticulitis, and irritable bowel syndrome. Also, many of these patients suffer from overly acid stomachs. Aloe, as was also found in Bland's study causes a substantial reduction in gastric pH. In other words, the aloe helps to reduce any excess acid in the stomach, something that can benefit us all.

The Anti-Inflammatory

The anti-inflammatory actions of aloe vera are attributed to a number of factors. The enzyme bradykininase helps to reduce excessive inflammation when applied to the skin, and therefore, reduces pain. Aloe vera also contains four plant steroids that are also important anti-inflammatory agents. Furthermore, aloe contains salicylic acid, which is an aspirin-like compound, possessing anti-inflammatory and antibacterial properties.

These anti-inflammatory properties of aloe are partly responsible for the excellent results on the gastrointestinal tract. The gel forms a lining in the digestive tract that has shown to linger for up to forty-eight hours. It also encourages correct pH (acid-alkaline) balance of the alimentary canal and soothes the internal tissues. Aloe vera, therefore, can help relieve colitis, ulcers, *Candida albicans,* and Crohn's disease.

Immune Strengthener

It is glucomannan, the major compound in aloe vera, that is mainly responsible for the immune-stimulating properties of the plant. This is accomplished by the increased activity of special white blood cells called macrophages that engulf bacteria and debris. This action helps protect and detoxify the body. The macrophages are also triggered to secrete chemical messenger substances, which stimulate other parts of the immune system. Noted research was conducted on the effects of glucomannan in aloe on human white blood cells. This renowned study, reported in the *Journal of Immuno Pharmacology,* concluded that aloe is an important immune system enhancer because of the high glucomannan content.[42] In addition, an article titled "Immune Enhancing Effects of Aloe," by Dr. J. C. Pittman in 1992, cited that aloe's glucomannan has a direct effect on the immune system, activating and stimulating macrophages, monocytes, antibodies, and T cells.[43]

The Healer

Aloe vera has a marked impact on the healing of damaged cell tissue. Glucomannan is also the main ingredient responsible for aloe's moisturizing and healing attributes. This glucomannan, along with other aloe constituents, accelerates the healing of injured surfaces. The presence of prostaglandins and essential fatty acid compounds within aloe vera was a surprising discovery. Aloe vera has the natural ability to convert essential fatty acids to prostaglandins (health protectors). This conversion for a plant is quite rare, but very lucky for us. The major essential fatty acid in this plant is gamma-linolenic acid. This acids exerts considerable influence on wound healing and anti-inflammation in the body.[44] The presence of fatty acids may therefore be another important biochemical component of aloe vera's wound-healing abilities.

Aloe vera also speeds up tissue regeneration by stimulating fibroblasts, cells that are widely distributed in connective tissue and responsible for the production of collagen. Collagen strengthens new tissue formation. Plant growth hormones in aloe, gibberlin for example, aid wound healing as well, by increasing protein synthesis.

Menopause

The cooling, soothing, tonifying effects of aloe vera have traditionally been used for menopausal problems in India and Latin America for many years.[45] The reason for this positive therapeutic effect may be aloe's ability to moisten dried up cells and tonify deficient fluids. Menopausal women tend to be low in compounds and fluids that nurture the liver. When the liver is properly nourished and not overheated, this critical organ can help to deliver vibrant health. The liver, when healthy, should:

1. provide vital energy to all body systems by strengthening other organs, especially the spleen, kidneys, and stomach;

2. regulate digestive activity;

3. renew and purify blood;

4. assist the release of toxins and waste;

5. improve fat metabolism;

6. balance hormones;

7. nourish hair, skin, nails, ligaments, eyes, and cells.

Menopausal women tend to suffer from extreme liver fatigue. Many women have lived with tired livers for years prior to menopause, only exacerbating the menopausal symptoms even further. Sluggish livers will have an adverse effect on virtually every aspect of bodily functions. In my experience, if left unchecked, a woman approaching menopause could experience severe menopausal symptoms. Aloe in juice form almost always becomes an important addition to my menopause nutritional program and quest to build the liver.

A MULTITUDE OF BENEFITS

Aloe vera possesses antibacterial, antifungal, antiviral, and antiparasitic properties. It has been shown to be beneficial for the following conditions: arthritis, diabetes, tumors, digestive disturbances, constipation, hemorrhoids, hepatitis, ulcers, skin diseases, menstrual disorders, teeth and gum afflictions, and problems associated with the ears, nose, and throat. Applied topically, it is used to treat wounds, sores, burns, and scalds. It acts as a bitter tonic to the liver and the whole of the digestive tract. Thus, it enhances the secretion of digestive enzymes, balances acid in the stomach, aids digestion, and regulates sugar and fat metabolism.[46]

Moreover, aloe has a generally "cooling" and "moistening" effect on the organs, and can be used for problems associated with excess heat and inflammation, such as fevers, gastritis, hepatitis, swollen glands, and herpes.[47] Specifically, aloe has a cooling effect on "hot" or tired livers. So symptoms such as headaches, irritability, and depression, almost always connected to poor liver function, should improve. It also might be beneficial for high blood pressure, thyroid imbalance, kidney stones, shingles, cold sores, warts, and fungal infections such as athlete's foot. Because of its immune-boosting and cleansing properties, it's an ideal remedy that can be taken long term for the maintenance of general health.

Finally, you need not take my word for it when it comes to aloe. There are literally hundreds of credible studies conducted at major medical schools, under internationally acclaimed researchers, reported in renowned scientific journals. So here are just a few more examples of such sound studies, supporting the benefits of aloe vera.

Peptic Ulcers: Aloe's effectiveness in the treatment of peptic ulcers was analyzed and reported in *The Journal of The American Osteopathological Society.* Twelve months into the study, patients demonstrated complete recovery after ingesting 1 tablespoon daily of aloe vera gel. This study concluded that aloe vera gel is an effective demulcent. Demulcents heal and prevent pathogenic irritants from penetrating ulcerous areas.[48] It has been suggested that the aloe gel inhibits gastric acid secretion, possibly through the presence of magnesium lactate.[49] This action further prevents and treats peptic ulcers.

Diabetes: Convincing results on aloe's antidiabetic activity have been investigated. Forty-nine diabetic participants enrolled in the study at the Mahidol Medical University and Hospital, Bangkok, Thailand. The subjects were given 1 tablespoon of aloe vera juice, twice daily in the morning and before bedtime. Blood sugar levels normalized and triglyceride levels reduced after only two weeks.[50]

Leg Ulcers: Aloe vera gel was successfully used topically in a study involving a small number of patients with chronic leg ulcers. The gel was applied to the ulcers on gauze bandages. A rapid reduction in ulcer size was noted, while two-thirds of the patients had complete relief.[51]

Cancer: The efficacy of aloe's potent immunostimulant glucomannan has been approved for veterinary use in injectable form for fibrosarcomas and feline leukemia. (Typically, 70 percent of cats will die within eight weeks of diagnosis of the diseases.) In this study, forty-four cat patients were injected with 2 mg of glucomannan weekly for six weeks, and reexamined six weeks after termination of the treatment. There was no control group, as owners were desperate to save their pets. Seventy-seven percent or twenty-nine cats were alive and in good health at the end of the twelve-week study.[52] The glucomannan from aloe was credited with significant antiviral, immunostimulant, and bone marrow-stimulating properties. Aloe researcher Dr. Plaskett points out that the immune-enhancing properties of the plant could benefit human immune response.[53] Patients with a history of antibiotic abuse or sluggish organ function, or those who have undergone surgical removal of tonsils, adenoids, or appendix, making them more prone to infection, should benefit. I usually prescribe aloe with other nutrients and herbs like cat's claw, astragalus, propolis, and vitamin C to stimulate immune response.

Please note that as a practitioner, I would never treat a cancer patient at the exclusion of conventional therapies. I have included this information for the purposes of cancer prevention rather than treatment. In addition, as a clinician, I made it a rule to never treat cancer itself; it is not my area of expertise. Others have spent a lifetime studying complementary treatments for cancers. At the clinic, if we see patients arrive with cancer, we merely try to help their immune response. If your immune response is strong, then you reduce your risk of cancer and degenerative diseases.

AIDS: Several studies have been carried out on the antiviral activity of the immune-enhancing compounds (mannan or glucomannan) with aloe. Glucomannan has demonstrated antiviral activity against HIV-1, influenza virus, and measles virus. Researchers believe that the glucomannan's main function seems to be its ability to enhance the action of AZT, thus reducing the amount of AZT required by up to 90 percent. Participants were receiving oral dosages of 800 mg daily.[54] White blood cells exposed to the glucomannan of aloe showed that it offered some protection to blood cells under attack.[55] This study certainly concluded with no cure for AIDS, but it does offer some hope. Perhaps just as importantly, it confirms the antiviral activity of aloe, which has many implications for all of us in our daily lives.

To summarize, this whole leaf from the aloe plant is healing to all organs and cell tissue. Assisting digestion, its compounds can relieve intestinal stagnation. Fungal infections, parasites, and bacteria are reduced. Aloe's unique properties reduce inflammations and help to repair damaged tissue. Its immune-stimulating and antiviral compounds are impressive, and its ability to nurture the liver helps to promote the free flow of energy through all meridians. It truly is the ultimate healer and strengthener.

USING ALOE

Aloe can taste quite palatable when mixed in fruit juice: that is, $\frac{1}{4}$ glass of aloe juice added to $\frac{3}{4}$ glass of apple juice can be both tasty and soothing. For those with obvious intestinal problems, $\frac{1}{4}$ glass of the aloe juice (with apple juice) twice daily, morning and evening, is recommended.

Aloe is easiest to obtain in juice form, gel, or tablets. Your local health food shop or chemist will most likely carry a selection of aloe juices. Follow directions on labels, as aloe concentrations vary with different brands.

I encourage people to keep an aloe plant in their kitchens. Use it in emergencies for minor cuts, scalds, or burns. Cut off one thick leaf and squeeze gel on to the injury; the gel will form a quick protective, cool coating, easy to wash off. Its healing compounds will absorb into the pores. It's easy to grow in a pot that drains well but will not tolerate temperatures below 40°F. It likes sun, but not direct, burning sunlight; a nice bright window will do nicely.

ALOE SELF-ANALYSIS

Do you recognize yourself?
If you suffer from one or more of the following symptoms, then you may need aloe vera.

Inflammatory Conditions

❏ Burns

❏ Scalds

❏ Sores

❏ Fever

❏ Swollen glands

❏ High blood pressure

Bowel Conditions

❏ Constipation (that is, fewer than 1–2 bowel movements daily or hard, rabbit-like stools)

❏ Irritable bowel syndrome

❏ Diverticulitis

❏ Colitis

Digestive Conditions

❏ Stomach ulcers

❏ Burping

❏ Bloating

❏ Gas

Other

❏ Yeast or fungal related problems (e.g., athlete's foot, thrush, *Candida albicans*)

❏ Diabetes

❏ Thyroid imbalance

❏ Immune dysfunction

Depending on the severity of the condition, you may need aloe vera on a short- or long-term basis. Dosage requirements may vary. Follow recommendations on the bottle and get the advice of a health practitioner.

7.

GREEN BARLEY GRASS:
Toxin Terminator

NUTRITIONALLY:

extraordinarily high in the antioxidant superoxide dismutase (SOD).
Also contains as much usable protein as meat.

PHYSIOLOGICALLY:

supports heart, lungs, liver, arteries, joints and bones. Fights free
radicals (unstable, dangerous molecules).

BENEFITS:

improves energy levels, stamina, and endurance. The SOD protects
cell tissue and removes pollutants, radiation, chemicals, metals, and
other foreign substances from the body.

Green barley grass is the only vegetation on earth that can nourish an animal from birth to old age, single-handed. Grasses have the extraordinary
ability to transform inanimate elements from soil, water, and sunlight into
living cells.[56] Our distant ancestors ate many grasses and raw foods; their
digestive tracts were designed to break down and convert it into living tissue. Gradually, humans began to cook the harder part of plants to make
them softer to eat. But it was not until the twentieth century that we began
to process our food with chemicals. And in the twenty-first century,
humankind is now genetically modifying some foods. All of these processes refine the nutrients out of our foods. As a result, new degenerative diseases continue to appear: heart disease, high blood pressure, hardening of
the arteries, heavy metal toxicity, and various cancers.[57]

While many of these processed foods are devoid of nutrients, barley grass contains every nutrient required by humans, except vitamin D, which is made in the skin. Scientist Dr. Yoshihide Hagiwara, once director of Japan's largest pharmaceutical company, says that plants have the greatest capacity to harness, preserve, and use energy from the sun for growth. Barley grass is one of the best examples of this power.[58]

Barley grass has as much protein as meat, but in an easily digestible form, and is crammed with vitamins, minerals, amino acids, enzymes, and chlorophyll. It has been reported to contain biologically active substances such as antioxidants and anticarcinogens.[59] This living green provides extraordinary amounts of superoxide dismutase (SOD), the key antioxidant enzyme that clears radiation, chemicals, pollutants, and other toxins from our cells. Barley grass is beneficial for all tissues and organs, especially the heart, lungs, arteries, joints, and bones. And while most grains and cereals are grown using herbicides, insecticides, and fungicides, which may contribute to cancer and other diseases, barley grass can easily be grown without them.

IN THE BEGINNING

Anthropologists know that early man lived on the rich variety of grasses that grew on the lush savannahs of Africa. As societies developed, so did agriculture, and the first crops to be cultivated were barley, wheat, rye, and millet. All cereal grains start out as short grasses—cereal grass. In its youth, barley grass is a deep green leafy plant with nutrient and molecular structure similar to that of green leafy vegetables rather than of grain, and with many times the level of vitamins, minerals, and proteins. The young germinated plant is like a factory of enzyme and growth activity. Photosynthesis in the green leaves produces simple sugars, which are transformed into proteins, carbohydrates, and fats.[60] The scientists who discovered the vitamins and nutrients necessary for human life in the 1930s found that giving green foods to their test animals often produced dramatic growth and vigorous health.[61] As a result, cereal grasses were investigated and found to contain at least carotene, vitamin K, vitamin C, and the B vitamins.[62]

"EAT YOUR GREENS"

"Eat your greens!" Does that sound familiar? For those without either time or inclination to devour green vegetables, dehydrated barley grass is convenient and one of the most nutritious natural substances. A 5-gram teaspoon is equivalent to 100 grams (4 oz) of vegetables like raw spinach, green beans, or lettuce. Barley grass contains all the known minerals and trace elements, a balanced range of vitamins and hundreds of enzymes for digestion. It has eleven times the calcium of cows' milk, five times the iron of spinach, and seven times the amount of vitamin C and bioflavonoids as orange juice![63] The small molecular proteins in it can be absorbed directly into the bloodstream. On top of this, it's rich in therapeutic chlorophyll. The structure of the chlorophyll molecule in the barley grass is nearly identical to our own blood molecules. When we eat or drink chlorophyll-rich barley grass, our bodies are being revitalized with new life and energy.

The Chlorophyll Within

Chlorophyll is the pigment constituent that makes barley grass and all plants the color green. The therapeutic elements have been scientifically researched for years. Here are a few of the findings. First, the chlorophyll in barley grass can reduce free-radical activity. Not only has chlorophyll been found to be efficacious for building hemoglobin in blood, but it's effective in detoxification, deodorization, and wound healing. Chlorophyll protects against toxic chemicals and radiation. In 1980, Dr. Chiu Nan Lai at the University of Texas Medical Center reported that extracts of cereal (barley) grass inhibited the cancer-causing effects of two carcinogens. Laboratory tests have shown that chlorophyll limits the growth of many types of viruses and germs, stimulates repair of damaged tissues, and inhibits the growth of bacteria. Finally, chlorophyll promotes regular bowel movements and reduces offensive body and breath odors.[64]

SO MANY BENEFITS

"Let food be your medicine" said Hippocrates some 2,400 years ago. What better medicine than barley grass—among the richest sources of nutrients available to humans.[65] The health advantages of barley grass are many:

1. It helps protect against pollutants, radiation, cancer, ulcers and digestive problems.[66]

2. It provides immediate energy for fatigued body systems by stimulating

the liver to release more stored sugar into the bloodstream, which then produces the energy needed by the muscles and glands.[67]

3. Nourishing the cell tissues with live organic nourishment from grass can have a powerful effect on strengthening the body's immune response against disease.[68]

4. Barley grass contains unique digestive enzymes that resolve indigestible and toxic substances in food. Studies carried out on the constituents of juice from barley grass revealed that various fractions of proteins and compounds showed significant antiulcer activity. The University of Tokyo found that barley grass contains antiulcer compounds that protect the stomach mucosa from injury.[69]

The SOD Factor

Perhaps most important, barley grass is very rich in the antioxidant enzyme SOD (superoxide dismutase) and the special protein P4-D1, both of which slow the deterioration and mutation of cells, treat degenerative disease and help the reversal of aging.[70] SOD, abundant in green barley grass, protects against free radicals—destructive scavenger molecules formed when radiation, bad air, chemical-laden food, and other toxins damage the body. SOD is either greatly lacking or completely absent in cancerous cells. Experiments show that P4-D1 can activate the renewal of DNA in cells severely damaged by X-rays or sun radiation. In fact, I advise my own patients to eat barley grass before and after an X-ray; and before, during, and after any air flight travel. (When we fly, we are subjected to a higher level of radiation, since we move closer to the sun.)

It has been well established that this superoxide dismutase (SOD) also has potent anti-inflammatory properties, more so than even some steroids such as cortisone.[71] A study conducted at the Science University of Tokyo examined the anti-inflammatory activity of green juice from barley grass leaves.[72] It was revealed that the anti-inflammatory activity of the barley juice was produced not only by SOD, but also by other proteins. Protein fractions P4-D1 and D1-G1 were isolated, and under further examination, both exhibited strong anti-inflammatory activity. During intravenous administration, researchers concluded that the barley grass proteins P4-D1 and D1-G1 exhibited much better anti-inflammatory action than the common aspirin.[73]

> **BARLEY GRASS**
>
> Green barley grass powder can be purchased from most health stores. You don't need much to make a difference. Please follow dosage directions on the bottle and mix in $\frac{1}{2}$ cup of water or juice (not orange juice, as it is too acidic). Tablets are also available. Once again, follow directions as outlined on label. I do prefer that you get the powder, if possible, as it is easier for the body to assimilate. Also, you'll need to take quite a few tablets to equal even just one teaspoon of the powder.
>
> For a change, alternate barley grass with one of the algae—that is, blue-green, spirulina, or chlorella.

Finally, the carbohydrate structure of barley grass contains large quantities of mucopolysaccharides, which strengthen all body tissues—including those of the heart and arteries—lowering blood fat.[74] In this age of fast food, we demand fast cures for our ills, many of which are caused by not eating a good, wholesome diet. I believe that barley grass—with its powerful array of protein, vitamins, minerals, amino acids, enzymes, and chlorophyll—is the smart, fast answer to remedy our nutritional decline.

I use barley grass in my practice because of its easily digestible form of protein and superior levels of naturally occurring SOD (superoxide dismutase). SOD is the key antioxidant enzyme that helps to clear the cells from radiation, chemicals, pollutants, and other toxins. To top it all off, barley grass is beneficial for all tissues and organs, especially the heart, lungs, arteries, joints, and bones. For those who are food sensitive, it is interesting to note that barley grass does *not* contain gluten, the sticky protein substance found in some grains. The biochemical makeup of barley grass and other cereal grasses is similar to that of leafy green vegetables and totally different from that of grains.

BARLEY GRASS DETOX JUICE

4 apples

2 pears

½ teaspoon barley grass powder

Cut the apples and pears into quarters. Purée the fruit in a blender or processor and strain the purée through muslin in a strainer. Stir in the barley grass powder and seasoning.

Simple to make with powerful health benefits.

BARLEY GRASS SELF-CHECK

Do you recognize yourself?

If one or more of the following apply to you then you may benefit from including barley grass in your diet

❏ Do you use a mobile phone?

❏ Do you use a microwave?

❏ Do you watch television more than two hours daily?

❏ Do you use a computer on a daily basis?

❏ Do you exhibit signs of premature aging (e.g., wrinkles, sagging skin, lifeless skin, hair loss, premature graying)?

❏ Do you suffer from degenerative illness (involving the heart, lungs, arteries, joints, bones)?

❏ Do you eat a diet high in processed, chemical-laden foods?

❏ Do you suffer from arthritis?

❏ Do you suffer from any other inflammatory conditions, for example gastrointestinal ulcers, hemorrhoids?

❏ Do you take anti-inflammatory medications?

❏ Do you live on a busy high traffic street?

❏ Do you live in a major city?

❏ Are you exposed to poor-quality air on a daily basis?

❑ Do you travel a lot by airplane?

❑ Do you spend more than two hours daily in traffic?

❑ Do you live within 60 miles of a nuclear power plant?

❑ Do you live within 200 miles of a nuclear military test sight?

❑ Do you live near electricity pylons?

❑ Do you have amalgam fillings?

❑ Are you frequently under the weather?

❑ Do you drink tap water regularly?

If one to three of the above apply to you, you may benefit from including small dosages of barley grass in your diet.

If from four to ten of the above apply, you may benefit from including barley grass on a regular basis. Perhaps, you could put yourself on a daily course of barley grass for a minimum of three months.

If from eleven to twenty of the above apply, regular consumption of barley grass for six to nine months may benefit you greatly. Dosage suggestions should be outlined on the label.

8.

FLAX:
Lubricating "Lube" Job

NUTRITIONALLY:

most abundant levels of omega-3 and omega-6 essential fatty acids, and in a perfect balance.

PHYSIOLOGICALLY:

lubricates bowels (colon); nourishes spleen, pancreas, and immune system.

BENEFITS:

helps regulate weight and bowel functions, lowers cholesterol, enhances skin tone, and improves immunity and reproduction.

I must tell you this one story on the subject of flax, from this very morning, ironically! Although I try to walk everywhere in the neighborhood for the exercise, I also regularly use a local taxi service for longer distance traveling across the greater London area. This morning, my taxi service sent one of their regular drivers who thinks he knows me a lot better than I know him. From past experience, I have learned that a brief excursion in his vehicle feels like ten rounds of the game "Twenty Questions." For our purposes, let's just call him "Harry."

As I sat down to enjoy the ride and sighed a sense of relief in honor of some quiet time, I barely heard some mumbling from Harry to break a much-cherished silence. Ignoring it to soak in the rapidly moving scenery, I heard it again. But this time his words were louder and definitely impolite to ignore. "You know, fish has more omegas than flax," he stated. "I beg your pardon," I said. "I said that fish has more omegas than flax seeds," he restated. The only thing I could think of was "Why was this invasive, somewhat jovial, but truly kind man, talking about flax on the same day that I was writing about it?" Did my little daughter color the word "flax" on my forehead before departing for her primary school? It was time to put a stop to this nonsense. "In all due respect, you're wrong, Harry. Flax seeds contain far greater levels of the healthy oils (omega-3 and omega-6) in a properly balanced and assimilable form," I explained. "No, I disagree," he argued. "What do you mean, you disagree? Have *you* spent years conducting clinical research, working with patients, lecturing, teaching, studying the omega oils in flax, obtaining worldwide data, compiling one of the largest private health libraries on the planet, and writing extensively on the topic?" I asked. Not to mention writing this very chapter on this very day. "No," Harry feebly replied. I wondered, "Are you a scientist, a biochemist, a botanist, or have you spent a lifetime studying food and biochemistry as I have done?" "No," he again replied. "So, where do you get such stuff? Where is your scientific authority?" I demanded. Harry proudly announced, "Oh, my wife is a doctor, a gynecologist by the way." "Is she a food specialist or nutritional biochemist as well?" I quickly retorted. "Um, ah, well, no, but she is a doctor," he offered.

Thankfully, we reached my destination. The car and the conversation came to a screeching halt. As I opened the door to disembark from this cigarette smoking, overweight, balding, part-time health guru wannabe and gentle but jocular man's car, I wanted to tell him that my second cousin-in-law's neighbor really does work at the White House in Washington D.C., and that qualifies me for Prime Minister, as his wife's gynecological expertise qualifies him for a dissertation on omegas. However, Harry was too busy mumbling something about flax to listen to my final thoughts. And for the record, flax is indeed better than fish as far as the healthy oils are concerned. I'm not saying you should not eat fish, but if you get picked up by my friend Harry, just remind him that flax is better than fish—and tell him I'm asking for him.

And speaking of taxi drivers and car rides, there is still one more quick, personal note left to say. When I lived in America, it seemed like everyone I knew used to take their cars every once in a while for a "lube job." After the "lube job" the cars always ran so much better, more efficiently, and the lives of these metal boxes were extended. My point is that lubrication definitely works. And I don't mean only for the car. The lubrication of our own body tissue cells, reproductive organs, hormones, glands, muscles, eyes, skin, hair, nails, joints, and bones is essential. That's what flax is all about, lubrication—a human "lube job" for the body.

WAY BEFORE LUBE JOBS

Way before lube jobs, the ancient Abyssinians were the first to use flax for food, roasting the oval shiny seeds before eating them. They were undoubtedly not familiar with the phrase "essential fatty acids," or acquainted with the benefits of vitamin E, beta-carotene, and fiber—all of which are crammed into these tiny seeds. In spite of that, they certainly knew a thing or two about nutrition and recognized a good food when they saw one.

Flax, also called linseed, is an annual plant with blue, pink, or white flowers, found in the Mediterranean region from prehistoric times. Fine linens made from flax fibers were found in the ancient Egyptian tombs. While Britons more recently recognized the virtues of its oil for grooming cricket bats, flax is now acclaimed in the Western world as an invaluable health and beauty food.

It is the fatty acid content of flax that makes it so valuable. Scientists have discovered that flax helps reduce blood cholesterol, lowers blood pressure, regulates weight, helps prevent colon and breast cancer, elevates mood, diminishes allergies, produces healthier skin, and enhances immunity.

Thinny Fats

Fats do have the most terrible reputation. In this era of low-fat foods and fat-free diets, the crusade against fats has gone mad. The most zealous campaigners even condemn oil-rich nutritious foods like nuts, seeds, and avocados. But no one can ever blame heart disease on avocados! I generally advocate nuts, seeds, and yes, avocados to my own patients. These oil-rich foods contain healthy fats—necessary in aiding weight reduction, lowering cholesterol, enhancing immunity, and even nourishing the reproductive organs, skin, hair, and bone tissue, effectively lubricating our bodies. These are the good fats—vitally important fats—necessary for life itself. And, believe it or not, these fats actually help you to metabolize fat.

Therefore, you lose weight! They are so important that they are called essential fatty acids (EFAs).

In my opinion, they should really be called *essential thinny acids.* That's how I refer to them in my practice, because my patients seem to like the "thinny" concept better. The new name seems to have a more positive psychological effect on patients making food choices.

Flax seeds contain the good oils, of which approximately 55 percent is omega-3 fatty acids. However, they contain more than just oil. Flax is an excellent source of high-quality protein and fiber. For example, $\frac{1}{4}$ cup (50 grams) of flax seeds has approximately 20 grams of fiber. Compare flax's fiber content with dried prunes (7.4 grams per cup), black beans (7.2 grams per cup) and brown rice (4.8 grams per cup). Most people do not get even halfway close to the optimal daily fiber intake of 30 grams. Good-quality fiber is a critical ingredient to ward off constipation, diverticulitis, colon disorders, colitis, hemorrhoids, cholesterol problems, high blood pressure, weight imbalances, and heart disease, all modern-day illnesses exacerbated by lack of fiber and poor dietary choices.[75]

Flax seed is unique because it contains both the essential fatty acids: omega-3 fatty acids and omega-6 fatty acids. Most important, it is the world's richest source of omega-3s. The typical modern diet supplies twice as many omega-6s as we need, but not enough omega-3 fatty acids. While primitive humans lived on roughly equal amounts, we now eat between ten and twenty times more omega-6s than 3s—a highly unbalanced ratio.

THE IMPORTANCE OF ESSENTIAL FATTY ACIDS (EFAS)

You need EFAs, but your body cannot make them; so you must get them through your food. Essential fatty acids are involved in systemic energy production and oxygen transfer. They maintain cell membranes, transport fats around the body, and are needed to make prostaglandins, the hormone-like substance responsible for stamina, reproduction, circulation, and metabolism.

Our cell membranes are made of fatty acids. These membranes are like the doors to the cells, controlling what goes in and out, thus facilitating communication between cells. EFAs help strengthen these membranes, making them more fluid and flexible. This speeds up healing and the building of new tissue. If you don't have enough essential fatty acids, then your cells use other fats to do the job. This makes the cell membranes more rigid and less efficient. Experts agree that unhealthy or leaky cells cause countless health problems: from allergies and cancer to a dysfunctional immune system. Thus, anything that strengthens the cell walls is critically important; EFAs do just that. Finally, essential fatty acids are involved in virtually every bodily function: the inflammatory process, the healing and repair process, the immune system, the neural circuits in the brain, the cardiovascular system, the digestive and reproductive systems, the body thermostat, and calorie-loss mechanism.

Omega-3 (Alpha-Linolenic Acid)

Omega-3s are primarily found in seeds and plants. Green leafy vegetables, cold-water fish (like mackerel, salmon, tuna, and cod), walnuts, canola, wheat germ, evening primrose oil, and of course flax seeds. Flax seeds contain over twice the amount of omega-3 fatty acids found in fish! In fact, flax seeds are one of the highest sources of omega-3, the healthiest of all fats, and contain more than any other food in existence. The increase in junk and processed foods coincides with the decreased consumption of omega-3s. Foods containing omega-3s tend to go rancid easily. Thus, in order to extend the shelf life of manufactured foods, processors often remove as much of the omega-3 components as possible. As a result, the customer rarely gets to consume these most healthy and important fats.

The benefits of omega-3 fatty acids are vast. Omega-3 oils help prevent and even reverse heart disease and diabetes, as well as inflammatory conditions such as allergies and rheumatoid arthritis. In 1982, Dr. J. E. Vane shared the Nobel Prize in Medicine for his showing how omega-3s help prevent heart problems. And Dr. J. Dyergberg, one of the world's leading authorities on omega-3s, studied the diet of the Inuit (Greenland) Eskimos, concluding that omega-3s reduce cholesterol, thin the blood, and lower blood pressure.[76] Omega-3s have also been shown to suppress tumor growth, improve immune function, and alleviate skin disorders, decrease inflammation, and help premenstrual tension.[77]

In my own clinical practice, I have found numerous benefits to patients, including smoother skin, enhanced muscle action, stronger cardiovascular performance, and better digestive function. In weight-loss diets, omega-3s may eliminate bingeing and food addiction, burn fats,

increase stamina, and possibly help overcome food allergies. It is important to understand that the ingestion of omega-3 fatty acids will not cause
weight gain. A study conducted at the University of Pennsylvania found
that these healthy fats help us to lose weight, or at least control weight. It
will be very difficult to lose any excess weight if you are omega-3 deficient. Thus, any weight-loss program must include these "thinny acids."

Case Study: Mr. Krauten, Bowel Problems

Mr. Krauten had endured a lifetime of problems with his bowels.
Movements were difficult, irregular, and uncomfortable. His skin had
shriveled, and its dry tone and texture screamed out to me, "Help, I'm so
toxic." Stool tests confirmed his toxemia and faulty fat metabolism. His
skin was always blemished with nasty-looking, large, angry pimples.

Eruptions will appear on the skin because of faulty blood cleansing by the kidneys and liver. These two organs must have the functioning strength to purify the blood. When they are overburdened,
toxins in the blood are excreted through the skin.

My program for Mr. Krauten emphasized foods to help purify the
blood and flax to lubricate the intestines and initiate proper fat
metabolism. Mr. Krauten desperately needed high sources of omega-
3 to correct his situation. (Yo-yo dieting in the past had included the
exclusion of all fats, including the good sources.) "I want you to
grind up three tablespoons of linseeds every other day and sprinkle
over a salad," I told Mr. Krauten. "On alternate days, I want you to
make my "Wake Up to Flax" recipe. Put three tablespoons of linseeds
into a cup of hot water, sit overnight and drink the gel and broth
only." (See page 81.) He reluctantly agreed.

I just saw Mr. Krauten the other day—after a six-month period of
flax powders and juice. The difference is quite remarkable. "Bowels
are brilliant" he said, "and my skin is as soft as a baby's bottom." He
can't believe the change. I must admit, he actually looked younger.

Results of an omega-3 rich diet and its use in the prevention of coronary heart disease on heart attack victims were published in the *Lancet*
medical journal. In trial studies, the effects of a Mediterranean-style diet,
rich in alpha-linolenic acid (omega-3) and antioxidants were compared

with a more "normal" diet with significantly fewer essential fatty acids, more saturated fat and cholesterol. After a first heart attack, patients were randomly assigned to a control group (303 patients) and the experimental group (302 patients). Heart patients were observed over a five-year period. After an average follow-up of twenty-seven months, there were sixteen cardiac deaths in the control group and three in the experimental; seventeen non-fatal heart attacks in the control and five in the experimental group. Overall, mortality in the control group was 20, but only eight in the experimental group, representing a two and a half times significant difference between the control group and experimental group. There were no *sudden* deaths in the experimental group. It was concluded that alpha-linolenic (omega-3) rich foods could help prevent coronary heart disease.[78] It was also reported in the *Lancet* that a diet that includes a high intake of alpha-linolenic acid (omega-3) has a beneficial effect on platelet reactivity in heart disease.[79] High platelet aggregation is associated with heart attacks. Therefore, if you have a personal or family history of heart disease, flax seeds should be a definite addition to your daily diet.

Omega-6 (Linoleic Acid)

Omega-6 essential fatty acids are widespread in our diet: they are found in nuts, seeds, grains, and most vegetable oils. Corn, peanut, safflower, sunflower, and, once again, flax oil, all contain omega-6 oils. But processed oils contain such a large number of contaminants and are so heavily refined that they are no longer good sources of EFAs. Only oils processed by cold-pressing methods are rich in these omega-6 acids.

EFA Deficiency

American medical researcher Dr. Donald Rudin puts another spin on this topic. He found that omega-3 fatty acid deficiency is a frequent basic cause of mental illness. Lack of omega-3 oils can reduce the number and size of, and communication between, brain cells, and can cause problems in learning, growing, and thinking. The brain consists primarily of these essential fatty acids. Severe deficiency can result in violent behavior, memory loss, anxiety, depression, and mental retardation. Thus, Dr. Rudin concludes that many diseases of the brain are caused by prolonged deficiencies of essential fatty acids, especially the omega-3.

THE SCIENTIFIC STUDIES

Flax seed can provide protection against some of our major diseases. Numerous scientific studies have been done proving its benefits:

- Flax seed is a concentrated source of lignans and isoflavonoids. In studies, these plant compounds have been shown to exhibit anticarcinogenic properties and have been associated with reduced cancer risk.[80, 81, 82] Flax seed consumption has, for example, been shown to produce positive biochemical changes in premenopausal women, which might lower the risk of breast cancer.[83, 84, 85]

- Research suggests that women with breast cancer excrete low levels of lignans, whereas women with no breast cancer history excrete high levels.[86, 87, 88]

- In Poland, a research project concluded that omega-3s from flax-seed oil were found to destroy cancer cells in rabbits.[89]

- A German study found that 30 ml of flax-seed oil daily for four weeks reduced the clotting agents in the blood.[90]

- An American study showed that a deficiency in fatty acids adversely affected the immune system.[91]

- Over sixty double-blind studies have demonstrated that flax-seed oil is very effective in lowering blood pressure.[92]

- Clinical research has found that some twenty-six diseases may be helped by omega-3 EFAs.[93]

- Canadian studies showed that bowel movements increased by 30 percent while flax seed was being consumed.[94]

THE BAD FAT SCENARIO

Too many bad fats—from poor-quality oils, fried foods, junk and processed foods, potato chips, baked goods, breads, fatty meats—disrupt our internal ear system and negatively affect the pancreas and gallbladder (the pancreas produces critical enzymes for digestion and the gallbladder helps to break down fats). Even people who are habitual fat avoiders will treat themselves with a bad fat "goodie." A body overwhelmed with bad fat and suffering from essential fatty acid imbalance may feel a dull ache or tenderness under the right rib where the gallbladder is located. Shoulder pain or a lost fourth or fifth toenail are additional signs of fat imbalances. Excess bad fat plugs the lymphatic circulation to organ function. The organ gets less oxygen and nutrients, then fails to function optimally.

The distinguished Japanese pharmacologist Professor Okuyama, speaking at the International Conference Society for the Study of Fatty Acids, stated that too much ingestion of omega-6 and low levels of omega-3 are contributing factors in the rise of Western-type illnesses such as cancer, heart disease, and allergies. He postulated that excessive omega-6 intake from poor-quality food choices saturates the cells with too much acid, causing inflammation and stimulating carcinogenic compounds. He concluded that many degenerative diseases are inflammatory conditions caused by improper ratios of fat in the diet.[95] A study published in *The American Journal of Clinical Nutrition* stated that our bodies must have both sources of fats, omega-3 plus omega-6, for optimum health.

While we should be eating an equal proportion of omega-3 and omega-6 fatty acids, in reality most people are eating far more omega-6 oils, and not enough of the omega-3. Once we can balance the ratio of omega-3 with omega-6, we will see a population with far less obesity and weight problems. The good news is that flax seeds contain the healthy oils (omega-3 and omega-6) in a perfect balance.

USING FLAX

Incorporate flax into your diet at least four times weekly. Purchase a box of linseeds (flax) or vacuum packed linseeds. Eat the seeds whole or grind them. Sprinkle them on salads for ease of use, two to four heaping teaspoons daily should ensure that you are getting a good balance of essential "thinny" acids. Linseeds are available in health shops; some supermarkets may stock them. Store them in the refrigerator.

The Conversion Catastrophe

Over the years in my practice, I have seen an increase in the number of patients who are not metabolizing fats properly. Constipation, liver problems, dry skin, falling hair, infertility, and infection seem to be on the increase, all of which can be linked to essential fatty acid abnormalities and conversion inadequacies. An analysis of patient food intake can often be quite revealing. It is important to know that the Western diet, high in junky, processed foods contain what are called "trans-fatty acids," or what I call bad fats. These bad fats are nothing more than altered forms of essential fatty acids. For example, many commercial oils are refined and exposed to tremendous heat in processing; translinolenic acid, an altered bad fat, is then formed. The body cannot properly use these bad fats. Worse still, bad fats block the critical conversion of omega-6, linoleic acid, into the favorable prostaglandin (PGE-1), an essential health protector for the body. These unfavorable trans-fatty blockers prevent the formation of healthy fats and accentuate the production of negative acids and unhealthy compounds that contribute to a host of problems. The most obvious are overweight and obese populations. But ultimately, the excessive ingestion of bad fats also leads to far more serious health ailments and degenerative diseases.

I frequently prescribe flax seeds or flax oil in combination with evening primrose oil or borage (starflower) oil for the high gamma-linolenic content (for the good fats). I have had exceptional results, particularly with women on gamma-linolenic acid. Many of my patients have managed their symptoms of premenstrual syndrome (PMS) as well as breast pain (mastalgia) with these good fats. This question of breast pain is much more common than most people realize. Mastalgia actually affects some 40 percent of women of reproductive age. And the reason that breast pain is as prevalent has much to do with this good fat deficiency–bad fat overage.[96, 97] When the fatty acid imbalance is corrected, the breast pain and PMS complaints disappear.

For all these reasons, I am happy to recommend that the best addition you can make to your life is flax. Get whole flax seeds. This way, you'll not only have the amazing healthy oils, and essential fatty acids, but the protein, fiber, and protective phytochemicals too. And all in a perfect balance. Simply grind the flax seeds in the food processor or nut grinder; 1 to

2 tablespoons daily should do the trick. Sprinkle them on salads, cereals, soups, pastas, stews, or anything else, and feel the beautiful energy from these tiny seeds permeate your whole being.

Flax (also known as linseed) is the most efficient form of essential fatty ("thinny") acids, because it has the most abundant levels of omega-3 and omega-6 in perfect biochemical balance. This specific form of fatty acids strengthens immunity and cleanses arteries. Flax nourishes the spleen and pancreas and lubricates the colon. It is excellent for tonifying the bowel and regulating bowel function.

WAKE UP TO FLAX

1 tablespoon flax seeds

1 cup of warm water

Mix the ingredients and allow to stand overnight. It will become soft and jelly-like.

In the morning, drink only the liquid. The flax will have soothing effect on the stomach and bowel.

DR. GILLIAN'S RAW VITALITY SALAD

Generous amount of arugula,
sometimes called rocket or roquette leaves

1 chicory (endive)

8 cherry tomatoes

2 organic carrots, shredded

1 white daikon (radish)

1 yellow squash

1 stalk celery

1 tablespoon linseeds, ground if you prefer

2 tablespoons raw sunflower seeds or sunflower sprouts,
sesame seeds or pumpkin seeds

1 packet dill seeds

Lemon juice or Algae Avocado Cream Sauce
(see page 131)

Rinse all the leaves and raw vegetables thoroughly with water. Tear the arugula and chicory into pieces. Peel the daikon. Slice the daikon and squash into thin slices. Chop the celery into bite-size pieces.

Place the arugula and chicory leaves in a large serving bowl. Artistically decorate the leaves with the red tomatoes, shredded carrot, white daikon slices, yellow squash slices, and celery pieces.

Sprinkle the seeds of your choice on the salad, and squeeze lemon juice over, or serve with Algae Avocado Cream Sauce.

Note: Raw foods are rich in live enzymes. Live enzymes assist digestion, assimilation, and absorption of vitamins, minerals, proteins, and other nutrients. These enzymes also break down unwanted fat, cellulose, and starch.

Arugula assists in energy production.

Tomatoes assist digestion and lower blood pressure.

Celery is high in the B vitamin niacinamide to promote relaxation, tranquility and even more restful sleep.

Squash helps cleanse key bodily organs.

Daikon eliminates congestion: opens the vessels for free flow.

Seeds assist in hormone production and health of the reproductive glands.

THE FLAX TEST

Do you recognize yourself?
If you suffer from one or more of the following symptoms, then you may need more essential fatty acids from good quality food sources, like flax seeds.

- ❑ Dry skin
- ❑ Ear cracks
- ❑ Weight problems
- ❑ Low-fat diet
- ❑ Premenstrual tension
- ❑ Miscarriages
- ❑ Chapped lips
- ❑ Rough skin
- ❑ Psoriasis
- ❑ Eczema
- ❑ Memory loss
- ❑ Thirst
- ❑ Poor attention span
- ❑ Constant cold infections
- ❑ Poor hair condition (dry brittle)
- ❑ Constipation

❏ Infertility   ❏ Confusion

❏ Liver problems   ❏ Thyroid problems

❏ Dizziness   ❏ Forgetfulness

If you exhibit from one to five of the above symptoms, you may have a MILD deficiency of essential fatty ("thinny") acids.

If you exhibit from six to fifteen of the above symptoms, you may have a MODERATE deficiency of essential fatty ("thinny") acids.

If you exhibit any sixteen to twenty-two of the above symptoms, you may have a SEVERE deficiency of essential fatty ("thinny") acids.

9.

PARSLEY:
Like a Multivitamin

NUTRITIONALLY:

the culinary multivitamin; a nutrient powerhouse. Contains high
levels of beta-carotene, vitamin B_{12}, chlorophyll, calcium, more
vitamin C than citrus fruits, and just about all other known
nutrients.

PHYSIOLOGICALLY:

restores digestion, supports the liver, kidneys and adrenal glands,
purifies blood and body fluids.

BENEFITS:

helps body's defensive mechanisms; chokes negative bacteria.
A great immune booster.

Parsley is just like an immune-enhancing multivitamin and mineral complex in green plant form. It is one of the most important herbs for providing vitamins to the body.[98] Parsley is made up of proteins (20 percent),
flavonoids (maintain blood cell membranes, antioxidant helpers), essential
oils, iron, calcium, phosphorus, manganese, inositol, sulfur, vitamin K, beta-
carotene, and especially vitamin C.

Parsley is a "warming" food, pungent with a slightly bitter, salty flavor.
It is moistening, nourishing, and restoring. In addition to providing essential nutrients, it balances and stimulates the energy of organs, improving
their ability to assimilate and utilize nutrients.

• Parsley enriches the spleen and stomach, thus improving digestion.

- It enriches the liver, thus nourishing the blood and body fluids.

- It benefits the kidneys and uterus and has a beneficial effect on the adrenal glands.

The high vitamin C, beta-carotene, B_{12}, chlorophyll, and essential fatty acid content render parsley an extraordinary immunity-enhancing food. If you want to boost your immune system, then parsley is the answer.

VALUABLE NUTRIENTS

Parsley contains particularly high levels of the following nutrients:

1. Beta-carotene

It is an adequate source of beta-carotene, which the body needs for the correct use of protein. This nutrient will benefit the liver and also protect the lungs and colon.

2. Chlorophyll

Parsley is abundant in chlorophyll, thus purifying and inhibiting the spread of bacteria, fungi, and other organisms. When tested in laboratory research, chlorophyll from parsley showed slight antibacterial and antifungal activity. Thus, it may be used to enhance immune response and to relieve mucus congestion, sinusitis, and other "damp" conditions.[99] A food that exhibits antibacterial activity can therefore aid digestive activity. Gastrointestinal organ function is not choked by negative organisms. Parsley may be used medicinally in cases of cystitis, since it has an antibacterial effect and the ability to flush out waste. Chlorophyll, high in oxygen, also suppresses viruses and helps the lungs to discharge residues from environmental pollution.

3. Vitamin B_{12}

Parsley contains traces of B_{12}-producing compounds. Such compounds are needed for the formation of red blood cells and normal cell growth, important for fertility, pregnancy, immunity, and the prevention of degenerative illness. The action of vitamin B_{12}, however, is inhibited by birth control pills, antibiotics, intoxicants, stress, sluggish liver, and excess bacteria or parasites in the colon or digestive tracts. Parsley helps to counter-act these inhibitors.

4. Fluorine

Fluorine is an important nutritional component abundantly found in pars-ley. Fluorine has an entirely different molecular structure from chemically produced fluoride. Tooth decay results from a shortage of fluorine, not flu-oride. It is the combination of calcium and fluorine that creates a very hard protective surface on teeth and bones. Fluorine also protects the body from infectious invasion, germs, and viruses.

5. Essential Fatty Acids

Parsley is also a source of alpha-linolenic acid, an important essential fatty acid that you now know from the previous chapter is too frequently defi-cient in today's diets.

THE THERAPEUTIC BENEFITS

Digestion

Parsley is an excellent digestion-restorative remedy. It promotes intestinal absorption, liver assimilation, and storage. A vast majority of people today have weakened digestive function and impaired toxin elimination. There-fore, any extra help in that area is a welcome addition. Because of its high enzyme content, parsley benefits digestive activity and elimination. The parsley root in particular strengthens the spleen, and can, therefore, treat malabsorption, bad breath, weight loss, loose stools, anorexia, and fatigue. It also improves the digestion of proteins and fats.

Liver

In the *Manual of Pharmacology,* physicians claimed that parsley is very effective in remedying liver disease.[100] It enriches the liver and nourishes the blood. Parsley helps reduce liver congestion, clearing toxins and aid-ing rejuvenation. Stamina loss and low resistance to infection point to a sluggish liver. This can manifest itself in blood deficiencies, fatigue, a pale complexion and poor nails, dizzy spells, anemia, and mineral depletion. In women, parsley improves estrogen and nourishes and restores the blood of the uterus. Conditions like delayed menstruation, PMS, and menopause (dry skin, irritability, depression, and hair loss) can often improve.

Kidneys

Parsley is effective for nearly all kidney and urinary complaints. It improves kidney activity. Parsley is not a treatment for severe kidney inflammation, but it can help eliminate wastes from the blood and tissues of the kidneys. It prevents salt from being reabsorbed into the body tissues; thus parsley literally forces debris out of the kidneys, liver, and bladder. It helps improve edema and general water retention, fatigue, and scanty or painful urination. It is an eliminant that I have even used in conjunction with complete nutritional programs to aid the dissolving of gallstones and in cases of gout.

USING PARSLEY

Fresh parsley is available from every supermarket in the country. Many even offer organic varieties of parsley. Parsley also comes in dried form as a seasoning. (A handful of fresh parsley two to three times weekly is a marvelous addition to any diet.) Parsley tea can be purchased from health food shops. If your digestion needs some attention, drink 2–3 cups daily. Nursing mothers should not drink too much parsley *tea* as it can dry up the milk supply. (Choose alfalfa leaf tea instead. It will increase the milk supply.)

Much discussion of parsley is anecdotal. Nonetheless, its nutritional content has been biochemically identified.[101] However, parsley's history of usage as a digestive tonic goes back to Ancient Greece and Rome, with its introduction into Britain in 1548. The chief researcher at Germplasma Resources Laboratory, United States Department of Agriculture, Dr. James Duke, discussed the use of parsley tea as an aid for dysentery and for the reduction of high blood pressure. The U.S. military then served it to troops in the trenches as part of a series of governmental experiments.[102]

In conclusion, parsley contains high amounts of vitamin A, chlorophyll, calcium, magnesium, iron, and beta-carotene, but most abundantly, vitamin C in an easily absorbable form. I tell my patients it's like a multivitamin in your food. I encourage people to use parsley leaves in food preparation and cooking meals. I use parsley in soups, stews, and casseroles. I simply throw it in at the end of preparation, just before serving the dish. In this way, the parsley is served raw but warm with the cooked meal. Parsley also makes for an excellent complement to any salad.

GILLIAN'S PARSLEY PEA SOUP

2 cups split peas (green or yellow)

6 cups water

1 vegetable bouillon cube; or 1 tablespoon tamari sauce

3 large carrots

2 red onions

2 medium potatoes

1 clove of garlic, crushed (optional)

1–2 generous handfuls of finely chopped fresh parsley

sea salt to taste

Soak the peas in water for 1 hour if you have the time available. You don't have to do this, but I've found that this makes the peas even easier to digest.

Rinse the peas and place in a saucepan. Cover with the water and bring to a boil. Reduce heat and cover. Simmer for approximately 1 hour.

Add the vegetable bouillon.

Meanwhile chop the carrots, red onions, and potatoes. Add these to the simmering peas for the last 30 minutes with the garlic, if using. Season to taste.

When the vegetables are soft, either blend entire mixture for a smooth, creamy consistency; or simply mash carrot against the sides of the pan with a large fork. Your soup will become speckled with orange color.

Add the freshly chopped parsley in at the end, once soup has finished simmering.

If you opt for the blended version, parsley can also be part of the blend. This makes it very easy on the digestion. Option 2 with freshly chopped parsley sprigs as a garnish is a tasty alternative. Add sea salt to taste if necessary.

CREAMY PARSLEY DRESSING

*1 handful parsley, washed and
rinsed and cut finely*

*½ cup water; or ¼ cup flax,
olive, or sunflower oil
(do not use too much water,
as dressing will be runny)*

2 tablespoons lemon juice

½ teaspoon sea salt

2 ounces soft tofu

Blend all ingredients until a smooth and creamy texture forms.

DO YOU PASS THE PARSLEY TEST?

To decide if you may benefit from including parsley in your life, ask yourself these simple questions.

❏ Is your digestion 100 percent perfect? (that is, no tummy problems)

❏ Are you completely free of all negative health symptoms—absolutely nothing to complain about?

❏ Do you live a stress-free life? (Stress rapidly depletes nutrients, weakening our immune systems.)

❏ Do you eat a daily supply of greens?

If you answer "no" to even just one of the above questions, then you can only benefit by including parsley. Use it in your choice of food as a "multivitamin" digestive aid garnish at least a couple of times weekly.

10.

SEA VEGETABLES:
A Mine of Minerals

NUTRITIONALLY:

highest digestible source of all minerals.

PHYSIOLOGICALLY:

alkalizes the blood, removing acid and toxic metals. Activates enzyme energies.

BENEFITS:

improves digestion and assimilation of nutrients, and assists weight management. Enhances mental energy.

We now move on to what appears to be the most frightening food of all: seaweed. The very name sends shivers down the spines of ordinary people. My brother-in-law said there should be laws forbidding foods like this. I would never, ever, utter the word "seaweed" in the presence of my own mother. It is the kind of food that fuels the healthy food skeptics. But really, it's just not that bad. The most difficult thing about seaweed (which I prefer to call sea vegetables because that sounds so much better) is not the taste, texture, nor appearance. Actually, the difficulty is simply the preconception. A patient once quipped that there should be an anti-prejudice society for seaweeds.

The reality is that sea vegetables can offer an unsurpassed complement to most meals for both taste and nutritional value. And trust me, you'll feel lucky that I opened your eyes to this incredible superfood.

MAGICAL MARINE SUBSTANCES

Sea vegetables, or seaweeds, are a form of marine algae that grows in the upper levels of the ocean, where sunlight can penetrate. They are found in coastal locations throughout the world. Sea vegetables are classified into three main groups according to color: reds, browns, and greens. The color depends on the spectrum of light exposure during photosynthesis. All sea vegetables contain the green pigment chlorophyll, but in some varieties, it is masked by other pigments.

In their natural state, sea vegetables contain 80 to 90 percent water. Once dried, this is reduced to 10 to 20 percent. Sea vegetables contain an average of 50 percent carbohydrate, 35 percent protein, vitamins A, B (including B_{12}, which is rarely found in the plant kingdom), C, D, E, and K, fiber, and a maximum of 2 percent fat. Their most outstanding feature, however, is their mineral content. Plants from the sea contain more minerals than any other food source—including calcium, magnesium, phosphorus, iron, potassium, and all trace elements essential to the human body. Some varieties contain ten times the calcium of milk, and eight times the iron of beef. Iodine, vital for the health of the thyroid gland, is also abundant. Because they are so rich in minerals, sea vegetables often act as alkalizers for the blood, helping to rid the body of acid conditions, also called acidosis. Symptoms of acidosis may include stomach ulcers, insomnia, headaches, gas, bloating, foul-smelling stools, bad breath, water retention, arthritis, and other more serious conditions.

Another interesting substance in sea vegetables is a colloidal carbohydrate called *alginic acid*. Researchers in the Gastro Intestinal Research Laboratory at McGill University in Montreal, Canada, reported that this alginic acid, once ingested, is able to bind with heavy metals such as mercury, cadmium, and lead in the body, carrying them out of the system.[103] Alginic acid has also been found to remove traces of low level radioactive material.[104]

Sea Vegetables in the Clinic

In my own clinical practice, I have successfully used sea vegetables on patients who were suffering from metal toxicity. Anyone living in the modern world, especially in an urban setting, is most susceptible to heavy metal overload. An excess of these metals can cause anything from fatigue and confusion to memory lapse. And some researchers have linked heavy metal toxicity to Alzheimer's disease. Nonetheless, the regular use of these essential sea vegetables may significantly reduce metal toxicity. These sea vegetables can be purchased in health food shops and natural food supermarkets. They are sold in a dried form in sealed packages. When you are ready to use them, rinse and soak them. They will become soft again.

Sea Vegetables in the Kitchen

Sea vegetables can be used to enhance the flavor of all kinds of meals, including stews, beans, grains, pastas, soups, fish, salads, and vegetable drinks. You only need one or two strips. There really is not a fishy taste, contrary to the preconceived notion. Generally, sea vegetables will enhance a savory or salty taste. I usually find that there's no need to add salt, or as much salt, when using sea vegetables.

Arame   Soak for 5 minutes.

Dulse   No need to cook. Wash carefully.

Hijiki   Soak for 20 minutes then rinse. Use very small amounts as it swells up enormously when soaked. $\frac{1}{4}$ cup dried will yield 1 cup after soaking.

Kelp   Usually ground into a powder, used as a seasoning or salt substitute.

Kombu   Soak for 15–20 minutes. If not soaked, it will take 40 minutes of cooking to become tender. A couple of strips will help tenderize the food and make it easier to digest.

Nori   No need to soak.

Wakame   Soak for 5 minutes. Cooks very quickly (2–3 minutes only!)

When making soups, I don't bother to soak the sea vegetable. I just rinse and throw it into the pot, letting it cook with the soup broth. When the soup is finished, I usually remove the sea vegetable. If I'm in a daring mood, I might then cut it into small bite-size pieces and return it to the soup. Hopefully, my family won't notice. And so far, I've been lucky. They all love my soups!

The following are two of the most important sea vegetables.

Nori

Nori is my favorite sea vegetable for its high nutrient content. It grows along the northwest coast of Japan, where it has been cultivated for over 300 years. It can also be found in the coastal areas of Alaska, Washington State, and British Columbia. In its natural form, nori may vary in color from olive green to purple or brown. Its leaves resemble hollow tubes; some are large and flat and others are ruffled. Because nori grows by the shore, the saltiness of the sea is diluted by fresh water rivers, rendering it mild in flavor. This makes it acceptable to the Western palate. Nori is sold in thin, flat rectangular sheets. There is no need to soak it. Use it to make sushi. I often use it as a midday "toast" snack. To toast nori, hold it over a gas burner for a few seconds, moving it slowly to prevent burning. It should turn dark emerald green. Use scissors to cut it into strips or crumble and use as a garnish for soups.

Nutritional Value

Nori contains 48 percent protein, approximately the same as meat and eggs. It contains as much beta-carotene as carrots, and also vitamin C (50 percent more than oranges), B_1, B_2, B_3, B_{12}, and vitamin D.[105] Nori possesses a broad range of minerals with particularly high levels of calcium, iron, phosphorus, and iodine. It is rich in fiber and very low in fat. Use it in your soups, rice dishes, and to make sushi. Occasionally toast it, cut it up, and eat it as a midday snack.

Therapeutic Benefits

Nori is the most easily digested of all sea vegetables. It also aids digestion, especially after eating foods that have been fried. You most definitely need this sea vegetable if you eat a lot of fried foods. Consumed regularly, nori has been reported to reduce cholesterol and high blood pressure due to its high levels of essential fatty acids. Because the energy from nori is directed inward toward the lungs and gastrointestinal tract, it can move mucus, phlegm, and catarrh out of the body. It has also been found beneficial for the treatment of goiter (swelling of the neck due to enlargement of the thyroid gland) and edema (water retention).

Dulse

Also known as *Palmaria palmata,* dulse is a red-purple sea vegetable with smooth, flat leaves. The plant itself measures about 15 to 30 centimeters in length and has a unique spice-like, nutty flavor. Dulse is native to the North Atlantic and is gathered from the coasts of New England; Nova Scotia, Canada; Alaska; and Iceland. Harvesting is carried out between May and October. The plants are picked by hand when the tides are low and left to dry out in the sun and wind. Dulse can be purchased in health food stores and natural food supermarkets. It is mild in taste and a good addition to salads.

Nutritional Value

Next to nori, dulse has the second highest protein content of all common sea vegetables. It also contains the richest level of iron of any food—150 mg per 100 g dry weight.[106] This makes it a good blood strengthener. Like nori, dulse possesses high amounts of vitamin B_{12}, with just half an ounce (12.5 g) supplying the recommended daily amount (RDA) of this nutrient. It is also rich in vitamins A, B_2, B_6, and E, and the minerals calcium, magnesium, phosphorus, potassium, and manganese. Dulse is 33 percent dietary fiber, of which 16 percent is the cholesterol-lowering soluble form.

In my clinical practice, I encourage patients to use dulse since it is also so high in the essential mineral manganese. Manganese is an enzyme activator, which means it can motivate more enzymes to release, thus improving digestion and supporting the spleen. Dozens of enzymes are dependent upon manganese for optimal activity. The enzymes involved in repairing, restoring, and revitalizing cartilage and bone, and forming connective tissues, cannot be produced in the event of a manganese deficiency. For example, when a patient suffers from arthritis, osteoporosis, joint pain, creaking joints, knee, hip, or ankle pain, I get them to use generous amounts of dulse or dulse powder. If a child suffers growing pains, I can usually alleviate them by prescribing dulse along with a mineral supplement containing manganese, calcium, and magnesium. With female patients, I have noticed a clear link between manganese deficiency and repeated miscarriage and/or nutritional infertility. In such cases, the dulse has proven helpful in conjunction with a complete nutritional program.

The physiological value of dulse was studied by the Department of

Food Chemistry at Tokyo University, Japan. The study focused on the cholesterol-lowering abilities of the sea vegetable and the isolation of the active substance. The result indicated that all green sea vegetables, especially dulse, markedly reduced plasma cholesterol levels in rats when they consumed diets containing 5 percent dried edible sea vegetables.[107] Nutrition researcher Paul Pitchford concluded that dulse has the ability to lower cholesterol, ease the herpes virus, remove toxins, and relieve nausea from motion sickness.[108]

Other Useful and Nutritious Sea Vegetables

Agar-agar

A clear jelly-like sea vegetable, agar-agar is sold dried as a vegetarian gelling agent. Because of its bland flavor, it can be used in both sweet and savory recipes. Very "cooling," it benefits the liver and reduces inflammation and other heat conditions affecting the heart and lungs. A mild laxative, it promotes digestion and carries toxic and radioactive waste out of the body. It is a good source of calcium and iron. Use it to make creamy puddings and delicious jellies. I use it to make a tasty fat-free, calorie-free dessert called "kanten," but my husband prefers "Gilly's Jelly."

Arame

Don't be put off by its brown strands and stringy appearance. Arame is high in iron and calcium. It contains compounds that nourish the thyroid gland. I love it best cooked with root vegetables like squash and turnip. It is supportive for the spleen, pancreas, and tummy.

Hijiki

Black, firm, and nutritionally rich, with an abundance of iron, iodine, and calcium, hijiki helps build bones and teeth. It is known in the East as the "bearer of health and beauty," as it revitalizes hair, skin, and nails. It expands in the stomach like fiber, helping to stabilize blood sugar balance and raised blood fats. High in niacin and vitamin B_2, it soothes the nerves and also acts as a mild diuretic. Hijiki has a stronger taste, but significantly aids in the assimilation and digestion of food.

Kombu

In the ocean, kombu—a member of the kelp family—can grow as long as nine meters. The Emperors of China have used kombu for centuries as a flavor enhancer and food tenderizer. If you soak beans with kombu in water, it helps to remove the gaseous substances from the beans, thus preventing flatulence. In other words, the kombu renders the beans more digestible. Because kombu contains such a rich supply of nutrients, it is believed to help conditions such as high blood pressure, rheumatism, arthritis, goiter, and anemia. It benefits the kidneys and adrenal function, and has an anticoagulant effect on the blood, is a natural fungicide, and relieves hormone imbalances.

In my practice, I will sometimes use kelp (Japanese kombu) in powder, capsule, or tablet form. Kelp tablets are especially useful for those people who are resistant to the inclusion of the actual sea vegetable in their diets. So if you don't like the idea of eating sea vegetables, you can simply take some kelp tablets.

I have found kelp to be useful in cases of obesity connected with thyroid deficiency. By helping to regulate the function of the thyroid gland, and restoring endocrine deficiencies, a person can expect to see positive changes not only physically, but mentally and emotionally too. The body's metabolism, metabolic rate, insulin, and antibody production improve. Consequently, the patient seems better equipped to ward off chronic infections. Although kelp tablets are especially useful when there is a thyroid deficiency, they are also beneficial when used for conditions such as arthritis, edema, anemia, high blood pressure, growths, prostate and ovarian conditions, skin outbreaks such as psoriasis and eczema, and yeast due to its antifungal properties.

Wakame

A diuretic, it also moistens and softens hardened tissue. It nourishes the female reproductive organs and purifies the blood simultaneously. But don't worry; it's fine for both women and men to use! Its active compounds help to support the liver and nervous system. High in calcium, wakame resolves phlegm and counteracts growths and tumors.[109] It has a sweet flavor. Substitute fresh wakame for lettuce in sandwiches. I promise it'll be OK!

SEA VEGETABLE SUMMARY

Incorporate small amounts of sea vegetables into your diet a couple of times a week. If you are a person with a "cold" constitution—that is, who feels the cold, feels chilly a lot, and has cold hands and feet—then cook your sea vegetables with a little ginger, and/or add additional herbs for warming energy (see page 139).

Seaweeds or sea vegetables are unique superfoods with an abundance of minerals and elements. Yet so few people I come into contact with have actually considered using them. When I suggest to patients that they start to eat seaweeds, I often get these really funny looks. No wonder. I can tell they think I've finally lost the plot. But when inevitably, after much convincing on my part, my patients try them, they are pleasantly surprised, and definitely feel the positive effects over the long term.

That's no surprise to me, as sea vegetables are important remedies for toxic, tired bodies. Their unique compounds help to perform biochemical changes in our blood that seem to address the ailments of modern society. Sea vegetables are "cooling" to the overworked liver, chelating to heavy metals to which we are all exposed (through amalgam tooth fillings or industrial and environmental pollution), softening to hardened toxic deposits and metabolic wastes. High in nutrients that influence the thyroid gland, sea vegetables are often incorporated into my weight-management programs; they improve the body's metabolism and water balance, alkalize the blood, and reduce excess stores of fat or mucus. Sea vegetables are an important source of viable nutrition in an ever-increasing toxic world deluged by packaged, canned, frozen, microwaveable, "boil-in-the-bag" foods. Unfortunately, these prepackaged foods are too often devoid of nutrients, enzymes, and filled with additives, colorings, preservatives, sugars, and a multitude of chemicals. Sea vegetables are free from all these nasty compounds, and that's why they are fast becoming recognized as an impressive source of nutrition, packed with much-needed minerals and vitamins.

USING SEA VEGETABLES

Experiment with the different styles of sea vegetables. Use them in your diet, two to three times weekly. Add ginger or warming herbs (see page 139) in the wintertime or if you feel cold.

NORI ROLLS

2 cups vegetable pâté or Algae Avocado Cream Sauce (page 131)

raw nori sheets

1 cup diced cucumbers

1 cup shredded carrots

1 cup alfalfa sprouts, clover sprouts or sunflower greens

1 onion, finely diced (optional)

sprinkle of fresh dill (herb)

Spread pâté or avocado sauce on nori sheets. (Nori sheets should be shiny side down.) Leave approximately 1 inch of nori sheet exposed at one end to help seal the roll.

Across the center, put a row of diced cucumber, then a row of shredded carrot, a row of sprouts and diced onions, if using, with a thin row of fresh dill.

Roll nori from the bottom, squeezing tightly. When rolled up, it should be nice and firm.

GILLY'S WINTER JELLY

3 medium apples, chopped

6 tablespoons of agar-agar flakes

2 cups of apple juice

2 cups of water

½ teaspoon natural vanilla flavoring

pinch of sea salt

¼ teaspoon cardamom powder (optional)

Place all ingredients in a saucepan, bring to the boil, and simmer for 2-3 minutes. Stir until the agar-agar flakes dissolve.

Pour into a dish and leave in a cool place for 1-1½ hours in order to gel.

GILLY'S SUMMER JELLY

4 cups apple juice

6 tablespoons of agar-agar flakes

½ teaspoon natural vanilla flavoring

pinch of sea salt

¼ teaspoon cardamom powder (optional)

1 cup finely diced strawberries

1 cup blueberries

Bring apple juice and agar flakes to a boil, simmer for 2-3 minutes, stirring until flakes dissolve. Add vanilla, sea salt, and cardamom, if using. Put the diced strawberries and blueberries in a bowl. Pour hot liquid over the uncooked fruit. Allow the mixture 1-1½ hours to gel.

You have an easy to prepare, delicious snack with lots of nutritional properties.

Variation: Add ½ cup of raisins to sweeten the jelly.

GREEN SAUERKRAUT

2 cloves garlic

2 heads of white cabbage, trimmed with outside leaves reserved

1 teaspoon ground dill seed

1 tablespoon kelp powder

Process the garlic and cabbage in a food processor with blade attached or chop into very fine pieces. Stir in dill and kelp powder.

Place mixture in a large bowl.

Put reserved cabbage leaves over the mixture, and cover with a lid.

Leave at room temperature for approximately 3-4 days to ferment. Fermentation creates lots of friendly intestinal bacteria and vitamin C.

Keep covered in fridge. Should keep for 1½ weeks.

SEA VEGETABLE SURVEY

If you can answer "yes" to just one of the following questions, then you need sea vegetables in your diet at least a couple of times a week.

❏ Do you live in a polluted environment (that is, car fumes, dirty air, industrial pollution)?

❏ Do you indulge in alcohol one or more times weekly?

❏ Do you have amalgam fillings?

❏ Do you eat a lot of pre-packaged food (that is, quick-fix meals, not freshly prepared)?

❏ Do you feel like you need more energy?

❏ Do you need to lose some weight?

11.

STEVIA:
Curb the Cravings

NUTRITIONALLY:
contains protein, fiber, complex carbohydrates, and vitamins.

PHYSIOLOGICALLY:
regulates and balances blood sugar levels.

BENEFITS:
suppresses cravings for sweets and controls appetite.

You are all going to fall in love with this incredible plant. Stevia is a sweet plant, much sweeter than sugar—but its sweet taste is *not* the reason I classify it as a superfood. Stevia has the ability to regulate blood sugar levels, suppress sweet cravings, and lessen hunger pangs, as it may be effective for those suffering from diabetes or hypoglycemia (low blood sugar levels). Stevia is excellent for stimulating mental and physical stamina, and it can even suppress the bacteria that cause tooth decay. On top of this, stevia has no calories. And all of this is supported by very credible laboratory research and authoritative clinical studies.

STEVIA'S ROOTS

Stevia comes from a shrub with green leaves belonging to the chrysanthemum family, growing primarily in the Amambay Mountains in Paraguay. Sometimes known as "honey leaf," stevia has been used in South America for over 1,500 years as a sweetener and a medicine. The Guarani Indians of Paraguay used it as a digestive aid, and as a dressing for wounds and other skin problems, as well as to sweeten their tea. Although the Spanish were aware of stevia since the sixteenth century, it was not until the 1880s that Moises Bertoni, director of the College of Agriculture in Paraguay, became intrigued by the tale that a small stevia leaf could sweeten an entire container of bitter tea. He set about studying the plant and published several articles in the early 1900s showing stevia to be nontoxic with significant therapeutic benefits and far superior to sugar. The first modern stevia crop was officially harvested in 1908. Plantations subsequently sprang up in South America. Today, it is commercially grown in South and Central America, Israel, China, Thailand, and the United States, where it is licensed as a food supplement. It is widely used in Japan— where extensive toxicology tests have been conducted and proven it safe—as a natural sweetener.

SWEET NUTRIENTS

Stevia contains sweet substances (glycosides) that are not metabolized in the body, and thus are eliminated without any calories being absorbed. Therefore, you'll be pleased to know that stevia is not fattening. Apart from glycosides, stevia also contains protein, fiber, carbohydrate, phosphorus, iron, zinc, calcium, potassium, sodium, magnesium, and vitamins A and C.

It is an herbal food with an impressive reputation for healing the body. Not only does it never cause blood sugar to rise, but it actually brings down raised blood sugar levels.[110] Unlike sugar, it does not spur the growth of unhealthy bacteria and yeasts, which can infest the body, causing serious problems.[111] Stevia alleviates the craving for sweet foods by balancing the body's blood sugar levels and avoiding the see-saw effect of hypoglycemia (see below). Thus, stevia may decrease the desire to eat fatty foods and control appetite. Some people have found that their hunger decreases if they take stevia drops fifteen to twenty minutes before a meal.[112] Reported in the *Journal of Medicinal Plant Research,* American scientists have discovered that stevia acts as a natural diuretic, helping rid the body of excess fluid, helps mental and physical fatigue, harmonizes digestion, regulates blood pressure, and assists weight loss.[113]

Other Natural Sweeteners

White sugar, fructose, and corn syrup all qualify as natural sweeteners, but none are calorie-free. Unlike stevia, these natural sugars can cause weight gain, tooth decay, and hypoglycemia. Common sugars contribute to indigestion, bowel disorders, even hyperactivity and attention deficit disorder (ADD) in children.[114] Conversely, stevia causes no such adverse side effects. Nor does stevia produce mucus in the body, as sugar does; nor does stevia encourage the yeast and bacterial infections, which feed off sugar. But most important, stevia helps to reduce cravings for sugar, as it brings balance to the blood. Thus, stevia actually has an opposite effect from sugar even though it is sweeter than the natural sugars.

HYPOGLYCEMIA AND DIABETES

Sugar itself is like a drug if you use too much. And don't kid yourself: most people today eat far too much refined sugar. Our bodies are just not designed to cope with the enormous quantities of refined white sugar in today's Western diet. Many patients I see are prone to *hypoglycemia* and *diabetes,* the two major forms of blood sugar disorders, which can deservedly be called modern day plagues. In fact, from my own clinical practice, I have found that one out of every two patients has either displayed hypoglycemic symptoms at some time in the past, or has been clearly diagnosed with hypoglycemia. The "over-sugarization" (to coin my own term) of the general population has resulted in a situation whereby at least 50 percent are at risk of hypoglycemia. Hypoglycemia can cause mood swings, irritability, depression, fatigue, drowsiness, tremors, headaches, dizziness, panic attacks, indigestion, cold sweats, fainting, and even alcoholism. The brain needs adequate blood sugar to work properly; but if blood sugar levels wildly fluctuate, it can lead to such a litany of adverse symptoms.[115]

When I was an undergraduate student at Edinburgh University, I had a dear friend who was studying to be a lawyer. He was a classic diabetic. He would frequently bypass lunch for a candy bar or some chocolate. Then, when his blood sugar levels went crazy, he would scramble for the nearest pub and drink himself silly. I only wish that I had known about stevia in those days. Similarly, I remember several years ago reading a piece in the newspaper about how the vast majority of prison inmates were either diabetic or hypoglycemic—with unbalanced blood sugar levels. Imagine if we could get stevia into the prisons—or, better yet, how about into the schools for our children. I have found that when the blood sugar levels are balanced, and other biochemical levels regulated too, patients usually report increased mental and physical stamina, and enhanced energy.

A study in Paraguay concluded that the herbal plant stevia had a positive effect on people suffering from hypoglycemia.[116] Twenty-five healthy adults were admitted to the study. Analysis was carried out using the "double-blind" method. This meant that participants receiving treatment did not know if they were receiving placebo therapy or the dried aqueous stevia extract. Results showed a positive reduction in hypoglycemic symptoms between six and eight hours after giving the extract to the patients. Successful studies were also conducted on diabetic patients as well.

Another study on stevia and its therapeutic effect on glucose tolerance was conducted and reported in *The Brazilian Journal of Medical Biological Research*.[117] Twenty-two healthy adult volunteers, both male and female, took part in the research conducted at the University of Sao Paulo, Brazil. Participants were not using any medication, showed no evidence of sickness, and were of normal body weight. Liquid extracts of stevia were administered to volunteers at regular six-hourly intervals for three days. Glucose tolerance tests, approved by the American Diabetes Association, were performed before and after administration of the stevia extract. A glucose tolerance test may involve ingesting a bottle of sugar water on an empty stomach. Blood is then drawn every hour, and blood glucose levels are measured. A fall in blood sugar levels in any one hour of more than 20 mg per deciliter, or a level at any time of less than 60 mg per deciliter, may be indicative of a hypoglycemic condition, and an inability to maintain normal blood sugar levels. In every period measured, including after overnight fasting, the blood glycemic reaction to glucose diminished after treatment with stevia.

Several other studies have been performed to evaluate the physiological mechanism of stevia extracts. Biochemical reactions produced by the stevia inhibited the mechanics of negative compounds.[118] These specific effects caused an increase in the body's utilization and management of glucose, thus ameliorating hypoglycemic reactions.[119]

Hypoglycemia is the medical term for low blood sugar. When blood sugar drops too low, it causes an overwhelming craving for refined carbohydrates. To satisfy that craving, more and more sugary foods are devoured, causing a see-saw effect of soaring and plummeting sugar levels.

This is why if you start to eat just one chocolate bar, you're bound to crave more. The sugar gives you that rush (not to mention the cocoa, caffeine effect), but the drop is never far behind. The best way to beat the sugar fix is to go "cold-turkey": no sugary foods or sweets for a month, for example. It's like trying to dry out from a drug habit. I'm not saying you should never treat yourself once in a while. But you need to do the following:

1. stay away from common sugars and sweets as much as possible,

2. support your system with live nutrient-dense superfoods to balance meridians,

3. use stevia to balance blood sugar levels and banish cravings.

If you experience constant cravings, you are probably eating incorrectly. Cravings are a sign that the body is out of balance. Blood sugar levels are too low. Too many overprocessed foods, high in salt or sugar, will cause you to crave more sugar. Overgrowth of yeasts will cause cravings, since such organisms thrive on sugar. Refined foods are processed in such a way that key vitamins, minerals, and fiber are removed. Thus, an excess of refined foods exacerbate cravings. For example, a chromium deficiency will cause you to crave sugar. More than 80 percent of chromium is destroyed in the processing of foods. And by the way, chocolate cravings are often a sign of manganese deficiency.[120] Stevia satisfies carbohydrate or sugar cravings by helping to regulate blood sugar levels. The point of all this is that stevia could dramatically reduce our risk of developing blood sugar disorders, especially hypoglycemia and diabetes.

For hypoglycemia patients, I may use supplements of amino acids, biotin, pantothenic acid, chromium, zinc, and manganese. All of these nutrients can be found in living sprouts and living foods.

Case Study: Mr. Farrow, 65, Retired School Teacher

Mr. Farrow was a long-term sufferer of hypoglycemia and depression. He was not diabetic but had been warned that he was heading that way by his general practitioner. His diet was a recipe for diabetes, loaded with added sugar, caffeine, and missed meals—the major contributing factor to his wildly fluctuating blood levels and black moods. "I've no wife at home to cook my meals," he confessed when I cross-examined his ludicrous choice of food intake. "What kind of an excuse is that," I replied. Of all the feeble comments of the day, "this one takes the biscuit." I solemnly scolded Mr. Farrow. Mr. Farrow was suffering from pancreatic insufficiency, low blood sugar levels, and drastic mineral shortages including chromium. He was guilty of consuming a vile diet; his negative food input was the catalyst for his ailments. Mr. Farrow had to change his life. To cut a long story short, sugar and caffeine went out the window; living foods, herbal infusions, exercise, vegetable juices, positive thinking, and stevia came in as the norm. Preparing his own food was a requirement that I insisted would help him as a patient. Initially, 1–2 drops daily of stevia became the aid to regulating his blood sugar condition.

I can now wholeheartedly report that Mr. Farrow became one of my most dedicated patients and follower of my living food movement.

Clinical Cases

Researchers acknowledge that stevia's plant glycosides exert numerous therapeutic actions in the human body. Some countries already are regularly using stevia to normalize blood sugar, and treat diabetes and hypoglycemia.[121] In the *Medical Review Journal of Paraguay,* other studies showed the beneficial relationship between stevia and blood sugar levels—with no signs of intolerance—when tested on twenty-four hypoglycemic patients. Similar results were achieved on diabetic patients.[122] Dr. Julian Whitaker, in his *Health and Healing Newsletter,* discussed clinical cases whereby stevia increased glucose tolerance and decreased blood sugar levels.[123] In my own practice, I use stevia on those patients with a real sweet tooth—the type of person who is absolutely addicted to anything with sugar. In almost every case, the patient reports either a substantial reduction in cravings, or in some cases, a complete eradication of the sweet cravings. Several patients pointed out that they were able to curb other cravings as well. For example, one man who felt he needed pasta every day suddenly didn't feel the need for it so desperately once on the stevia. He felt more balanced. When the blood sugar levels are regulated, our cravings for certain types of foods should regulate too.

OTHER BENEFITS

Stevia has other medical uses as well. A study from the Hiroshima School of Dentistry reported that stevia suppresses dental bacterial growth.[124] In other words, stevia helps fight tooth decay and cavities. Conventional sugar, on the other hand, feeds dental bacteria and often causes tooth decay. Taken as a mouthwash, stevia can prevent gingivitis and gum disease. It is used in some dental products and recommended by many Brazilian dentists to retard plaque.[125] Brazilians have known the benefits of this plant for some time; it has had a long history of use as a gastrointestinal tonic there, well before these dental studies.[126]

Tests have shown that stevia inhibits the growth of *Streptococcus mutans*.[127] This explains the successful traditional use in treating wounds, sores, and gum disease, as well as demonstrates why it benefits those susceptible to yeast infections. Japanese studies—including extensive toxicity trials—have found no anomalies in cell, enzyme, chromosomal, or other significant physiological side effects from stevia, according to Rita Elkins in her book *Stevia, Nature's Sweetener*. And in Japan, more than 170 metric tons of stevia were consumed in 1987 with no documented side effects.[128]

To conclude, the most important element about stevia is its documented ability to regulate blood sugar, suppress the desire for sweets, and lessen hunger cravings. Stevia is therefore most beneficial for people at risk of hypoglycemia or diabetes. To see if you might be at risk of hypoglycemia, take my Stevia Challenge on page 107.

USING STEVIA

Stevia is no longer available in Europe. However, it is widely sold and used in the United States, Canada, Japan, China, and elsewhere. It can be obtained via the Internet.

Stevia should be available in powder or liquid extract. A special herbal shop may be able to provide the plant leaves. You must follow dosage directions on the label. When baking or making desserts, 1–3 drops of the extract should sweeten 1 cup of liquid. Best to experiment with this and see what works for you.

STEVIA CHALLENGE

Is this you?

If one or more of the following apply to you, you may have a blood sugar imbalance or hypoglycemia, and therefore require stevia.

❏ Diet full of sugar

❏ Contraceptive pill

❏ Two or more alcoholic drinks daily

❏ Alcoholic binges (once a week or more)

❏ Confusion or forgetfulness

❏ Anger

❏ Temper tantrums

❏ Mood swings

❏ Exhaustion

❏ Shakiness before eating

❏ Constant hunger

❏ Eating binges

❏ Frequent indigestion

❏ Occasional nausea

❏ Blurred vision

❏ Insomnia

❏ Crave candy bars

❏ Crave sweets

❏ Diet full of junk foods

❏ Liver disease

❏ Frequent headaches

❏ Depression

❏ Premenstrual syndrome

❏ Energy slumps

❏ Tremors

❏ Ravenous cravings

❏ Tiredness after eating

❏ Anxiety

❏ Cold sweats

❏ Weak legs

❏ Irritability

If you exhibit one to ten of the above symptoms, you may have a MILD blood sugar imbalance.

If you exhibit 11 to 21 of the above symptoms, you may have a MODERATE blood sugar imbalance.

If you exhibit 22 to 31 of the above symptoms, you may have a SEVERE blood sugar imbalance.

12.

SUNFLOWER:
The Energy Booster

NUTRITIONALLY:

power-packed with essential fatty acids; vitamins E, A, D, and B complex; the minerals zinc, iron, calcium, manganese, potassium, and phosphorus; and lipotropics. Excellent source of protein.

PHYSIOLOGICALLY:

massages the intestines, tonifies the bowels, and ultimately pushes energy and blood to all meridians.

BENEFITS:

the finest energy "pick-me-up."

My first introduction to sunflower, more than a decade ago, was from a ninety-eight-year-old osteopathic physician and biochemist in Trenton, New Jersey, named Dr. Samuel Getlin. He was one of the first complementary practitioners in the United States, a pioneer in the field some seventy-five years ago. Although somewhat eccentric, as his office hours often went into the wee hours of the night, he treated many scores of people—including, by the way, the movie star Katharine Hepburn. One of the many concepts that sticks in my mind from this extraordinary man was his recommendation to eat sunflower seeds. "Whenever you feel hungry, tired, or wishing for a sweet, always make sure you have a few handfuls of sunflower seeds nearby. You'll be just fine then," he reassured softly.

Other doctors have recognized the medicinal powers of sunflower seeds as well. Medical doctor John Douglas recommends sunflower seeds to his patients with raised blood pressure, cardiovascular problems, and high cholesterol.[129] Scientists have also discovered that sunflowers, float-ing on the surface of highly contaminated water, have successfully re-moved toxic elements, including uranium, cesium, and strontium.[130] In one Russian clinic, a sunflower-seed tincture was used to treat malarial fever. It has also been used in Turkey, in cases where quinine and arsenic have failed to treat malarial fever, and had the advantage of being safer in the long term.[131]

But thanks to Dr. Getlin, sunflower in my practice is known as the "energy pick-me-up," due to its nourishing of the digestive organs, the spleen, and the enzyme-producing pancreas, and compounds capable of lubricating the intestines. The B vitamins and essential fatty acids gives the hormone-producing adrenal glands a wake-up call. The end result is a more biochemically efficient and energized you.

PACKED WITH POWER

The sunflower is a native of Mexico and Peru and was introduced to Great Britain in the sixteenth century. It was much revered by the Aztecs; in their temples, the priestesses were crowned with sunflowers. The Spanish con-querors often created images of sunflower in pure gold sculptures. The sunflower is the national emblem of Peru, and in Kansas, it's the official state flower. Sunflowers can come in over 100 different species. High oil type sunflower seeds are processed to obtain the oil and sunflower meal (made from grinding the dehulled sunflower seeds). The sunflower is a very versatile crop, as every part of it can be utilized. The leaves are used as cattle fodder; the fibrous stems are processed for paper-making; the flowers contain a yellow dye; and the seed is rich in a sweet-tasting healthy oil, more similar in flavor and composition to olive oil than any other vegetable oil.

Sunflower oil is high in polyunsaturated fatty acids, essential linoleic acid, vitamin E, and the nutrient choline. It has a protein content of 25 per-cent and is rich in the B vitamins (thiamine, pyridoxine, niacin, and pan-tothenic acid) and vitamin A. It has a high potassium/low sodium ratio, and significant levels of zinc, iron, calcium, copper, manganese, and phos-phorus. The vitamin D stored in the sun-filled seeds aids calcium utiliza-tion. Sunflower oil also has a high concentrate of lipotropic constituents. Lipotropic literally means "fat-mover." This term refers to substances that are able to assist the liver in metabolizing fats and removing them from the bloodstream. Lipotropes also aid the metabolism of fat-soluble nutrients and hormones.

Sunflower seeds and meal are a desirable source of protein and a potential substitute for meat. The protein is slightly lower in the amino acid lysine, but more than adequate in the other essential amino acids. Typical sunflower meal contains approximately 45 to 50 percent protein. The meal is superior in nutrient content to other meals. For example, sunflower has more concentration of B vitamins than soybeans, more pantothenic acid (B_5) than wheat germ, and so on. As a result, sunflower seeds are nourishing to the adrenal glands and adrenal function.

Poor adrenal function usually results in energy slumps, due to the inability of the adrenal glands to produce balanced levels of hormones throughout the day. Deficiencies of B vitamins, in particular pantothenic acid, can often be the underlying cause of poor adrenal gland function. Due to its positive effect on these important glands and its ability to strengthen function of the spleen and stomach, sunflower seeds can render those mid-afternoon energy slumps a thing of the past. Get into the habit of carrying sunflower seeds around with you as an energy "pick-me-up." These seeds are far better for you than a cup of coffee or some snack foods that simply give you a zap of sugar, and excess calories. Raw sunflower seeds are delicious and nutritious, with valuable sources of good quality protein and essential fatty acids, vitamins, and minerals.

Case Study: Mrs. Norris, 44, Typist/Receptionist

Mrs. Norris, from Ealing, England, was a caffeine addict. When she first came to see me for "tiredness," she was consuming a diet that I can only describe as abominable, with virtually no freshly prepared food. "Too busy," she sighed on my questioning her dietary habits. "Just give me something so I'm not so tired." Most of what Mrs. Norris was eating was laden with sugar and/or loaded with caffeine. Mid-afternoon chocolate snacks were a staple. She told me emphatically that "without her caffeine fix and chocolate goodies," she "could not get through the day." She would "be falling asleep at her desk." She was also under a great deal of emotional stress when we just met, raising her son alone with little help. Biochemical tests confirmed my initial intuitive feeling and the tongue and physical diagnosis. Mrs. Norris was suffering from poor adrenal function and nutrient deficiencies. With poorly functioning adrenal glands, you can experience a multitude of symptoms from midday energy slumps, bloating, unexplained hair loss, to insomnia, PMS, food allergies, insatiable cravings, and more. Everything from metabolism, energy production, blood pressure, immunity, menstrual cycles, and even feeling sexy, will depend on a well-fed, healthy functioning de-stressed adrenal system.

A rigorous adrenal-strengthening program was implemented to rebuild these tiny but powerful glands, which sit above the kidneys. Sunflower seeds, living foods, herbs, and nutritional supplements were used to feed the glands and eradicate nutrient deficiencies. It was not an easy transition for Mrs. Norris whose body was akin to a burned-out car battery with little "juice" left with which to jump-start it. Mrs. Norris eventually did recover, was weaned from caffeine, and no longer craved chocolate treats. Instead her midday boost comes from raw sunflower seeds. She informed me the other day that she is now growing her own sunflower sprouts and is experimenting with my seed cheese recipe. Obviously sunflower seeds alone did not arrest her condition, but they can go a long way to helping in the task of building the body as opposed to depleting it. Sunflower compounds specifically aid the organs responsible for energy production: the spleen, pancreas, and adrenal glands. They're definitely worth snacking on.

ENERGIZING THE ORGANS

Sunflower "warms" the body by pushing energy and blood up and out toward the surface. It strengthens the spleen and pancreas, two organs intimately involved in energy production. Energy can then flow more freely through the body systems to other supporting internal organs. Health problems occur when energy stagnates. For example, yeast-related illnesses, tumors, cysts, obesity, and cancers are all signs of energy block-ages and "damp" in the body. Compounds from sunflower "warm" you up, help transport the blood, and maintain the activity of key organs, preventing obstructions and damp accumulations. The seeds and oil have a diuretic and expectorant (drying) effect, and thus have been employed in the treatment of bronchial, throat, and lung infections, coughs, colds, and whooping cough.

Patients with scaly dermatitis and skin lesions participated in a study on the benefit of applying sunflower seed oil to the skin. Patients were previously shown to be deficient in essential fatty acids due to chronic malabsorption. They exhibited abnormally low levels of linoleic acid. After two weeks of application of sunflower-seed oil on the right forearms of the patients, a marked improvement was noted. The level of linoleic acid in the skin layers had increased and the scaly lesions had disappeared. No changes were recorded in the left arms after topical application of olive oil, rich in oleic acid. The application of sunflower-seed oil had a positive effect on the damaged skin.[132]

Sunflower oil lubricates the intestines, due to high levels of polyunsaturated fatty acids, and can be very effective in toning the bowels. Sunflower not only supports and strengthens the liver, due to its fat-absorbing effect, but also softens the stools, allowing easier and more effective evacuation. A study carried out in Sweden showed that a diet rich in sunflower oil lowered the level of harmful cholesterol in the blood.[133] The same study also found sunflower oil to be significantly more effective than olive oil in reducing cholesterol.

For all of these convincing reasons, go out and get some (raw) sunflower seeds. You can sprinkle them on salads, cereals, soups, stews, and desserts, even sprout them (really delicious), or just munch them as is, à la Dr. Getlin.

USING SUNFLOWER

Use sunflower seeds as much as you like. Carry them with you for a midday snack. A couple of handfuls daily or every other day is fine. Sunflower sprouts two to three times weekly would be a superb addition to your food intake.

Dr. Gillian's Living Sunflower Dream

6 carrots (with tops, if desired)

1 apple

1 ripe avocado

10 basil leaves

½ cup sunflower seeds or sunflower sprouts

1 slice lemon

Juice the carrots and apple through a juicer.

Blend the avocado, basil, and sunflower seeds in a food processor. Mix with the carrot and apple juice and squeeze a dash of lemon into the drink. Delicious!

Carrots: Improve liver function, eliminate putrid bacteria and wastes.

Tops: Rich in minerals. Bitter in flavor.

Avocado: Food for your brain; easily digested. Rich source of protein. High in minerals that build the blood.

Basil: Immune stimulant. Aids digestion as it benefits the stomach and related digestive organs.

Apple: Stabilizes blood sugar, detoxifies heavy metals. A food for the nerves.

Lemon: Gas buster! Alleviates flatulence. Liver stimulant.

Sunflower Mayonnaise

1 cup sunflower seeds (soaked)

1 cup Green Sauerkraut (see page 99)

1 avocado

handful of fresh dill

1 teaspoon dulse

Blend all the ingredients until smooth and creamy. Use as a tasty dressing.

Sunflower Seed Cheese

High in enzymes, B vitamins, and natural acidophilus. This recipe is a little time consuming but an absolute must for those who want to avoid dairy cheese and for those who desire a change from soy or rice cheeses. You will need a good blender and a cheese bag.

2 cups sunflower seeds

1 cup sesame seeds

½ cup chopped onions

2-4 tablespoons water

1 teaspoon miso (optional)

Soak the seeds for 8–12 hours overnight.

Combine all the ingredients in a blender for approximately 4 minutes.

After blending, pour mixture into a cheese bag, strain liquid off and serve the cheese immediately. The more liquid (or whey) you drain off, the firmer the cheese will be.

To ferment and create more natural acidophilus:

Pour mixture into a bowl, cover with a cloth. Let mixture stand 6–8 hours. Spoon into a cheese bag. Store in the fridge overnight. Keep a bowl underneath the bag to catch the liquid seeping from bag.

The following variations of the basic recipe can be fun to try:

Spicy Cheese

Add 1 teaspoon fresh cayenne.

Blend with ginger, 2 cloves garlic, ¼ cup fresh basil, dulse, and oregano to taste.

Red Cheese

Add 1 beetroot and 1 red pepper.

Green Cheese

Add:

½ cup fresh parsley

1 green pepper

½ cup basil leaves

1 tablespoon dulse (optional)

Blend with ginger and $\frac{1}{2}$ cup finely chopped onions. Substitute sesame seeds with pumpkin seeds.

SUNFLOWER CHECK

Do you need them?
If you suffer from one or more of the following symptoms, then you may benefit from including sunflower seeds in your diet.

❑ Allergies

❑ Mid-afternoon energy slump

❑ Constant tiredness

❑ Spare tire, difficulty shifting weight even when exercising

❑ Mood swings/depression

❑ Cravings for bread, salt, or sweets

❑ Difficulty getting out of bed in the morning

❑ Apathetic

❑ Prolonged stress

❑ Insomnia/lack of sleep

❑ Light-headed, feeling faint

❑ Hungry all the time

❑ Low blood pressure

If you exhibit one to three of the above symptoms, incorporate more sunflower seeds and sprouts into your life.

If you exhibit four to eight of the above symptoms, use sunflower along with other living foods on a daily basis. You may be suffering from poor adrenal function (see page 110).

If you exhibit more than eight of the above symptoms, you must include sunflower seeds and sprouts in your life; please investigate (with the help of a practitioner) your adrenal function (see page 110).

13.

WILD BLUE-GREEN ALGAE:
The Harmonizer

NUTRITIONALLY:

contains virtually every nutrient known to man in a most absorbable and balanced form. Particularly high in assimilable protein, amino acid peptides, digestible minerals, active enzymes and pigments.

PHYSIOLOGICALLY:

harmonizes physiological and biological human functions. Supports virtually every system. Builds the blood.

BENEFITS:

helps you to think better, improves memory. Strengthens immunity, and provides a feeling of well-being, vigor, and vitality. Helps prevent unhealthy bacteria, pathogens, fungi, viruses, colds, and flu. Removes excess mucus.

In 1997 I wrote a small book, *The Miracle Superfood: Wild-Blue-Green Algae,* which has been well received in various parts of the world, including the United States. Last year, more than 5,000 Americans lined up in the Minnesota capital city, Minneapolis, at the largest conference hall to obtain autographs on their copies of my book. And for good reason: this small, but important book tells the sobering story of my years of personal experience, scientific studies, and clinical research on this essential algae.

About fifteen years ago while hosting the *Healthline Across America* radio show from New York, a special guest came on the program. This special guest was a man in his mid-forties who wanted to share with my audience his successful fight against the most insidious strain of leukemia. He had been free of the disease for more than ten years. Prior to the ten years, he had faced two relapses of leukemia, and a third relapse would have been considered fatal. Frankly, we now know that generally a second relapse is also frequently fatal. Nonetheless, after his second relapse, this man walked out of hospital (something I do not condone). He decided to make radical changes to his lifestyle, and then hope for the best. He moved "from the busy metropolis of Chicago to the quiet, less polluted backwoods of Maine."

Somehow, with the grace of God, "the leukemia disappeared, never to return again." I could feel my radio audience gripped by his words, his story. And then my question came: "The national statistics tell us that most people in your situation would never have made it. Some 90 percent die within three years from AML-leukemia. You have been fine for the past ten. Is there anything you're doing differently that you feel is keeping you alive?" The air went silent. In radio, a few seconds of blank space feels like a tense eternity, especially when millions of people are listening. I could feel the sweat on my neck, waiting for his answer. Finally, "Well, yes," he blurted. "Yes what?" I queried with trepidation, realizing that at least he had answered. "Yes, there is something that I have been doing every day for the past ten years without fail, since I walked out of that hospital." "What is that?" I cautiously asked. "A couple days after I left hospital to start my new life, a wise man told me to start taking wild blue-green algae. I had never even heard of it." Neither had I, by the way. He continued, "So I started to take it every single day. And I never miss it. In the past ten years, I have taken this algae every single day, and the leukemia is gone and I have not had a relapse since. In fact, I am very healthy now. I feel this algae was sent to me by an angel, God's food." The audience got what it wanted, and so did I. His story changed my life as well. I then made it my life mission to learn everything that I possibly could about this algae. I would spend more than a decade or so researching this one superfood, even writing a doctoral dissertation on it, and then a book.

GOD'S PLAN

But it's funny how life goes. About two years after interviewing this leukemia-healed man, my own beautiful nephew, Erik, was diagnosed at the age of twelve with the same exact strain, AML-leukemia. He died the next year at thirteen. He was resistant to my ways, but he must have known God's plan for himself. Interestingly enough, less than two years after Erik died, a lovely Scottish couple appeared at my clinic doorstep with yet another beautiful twelve-year-old child, a girl. The mum was in tears; the dad's eyes red; and the daughter with a look of fear, yet calm. Their daughter had survived one relapse of leukemia. The hospital doctors were very worried; their prognosis was not good, to say the least. Mum and dad were terrified and justifiably sad. I thought to myself, "What could I possibly do? It's now in God's hands." These people had too much expectation of me. They had read some feature about me in a Scottish newspaper—something like "local girl makes good"—and their hope was being pinned on that story.

I was scared. After all, I was not able to save Erik. So why should I be able to save someone else? The raw grief from the death of my young nephew and the pain and agony of his mum losing her only child were still eating at me. Now a new set of parents, from my own homeland, came to me to save their only child. The parallels were too coincidental for my taste. As these parents and their beautiful child left my office, I began to tremble; then weeping and downright wailing. It was all just too close to home. And then I allowed the light to penetrate me, or shall I say "I saw the light." Was this some chance of vindication? Redemption? Renewal? Erik was gone, but this wee girl's fate could be different. There must have been a reason that these people were sent to me. Now was my chance to share the information and hope that it would be received.

This time, however, I would not stand for petty resistance, skepticism nor cynicism as in the case of my nephew. So I told this little girl that in order to be my patient she would have to literally obey and implement everything that I told her. I didn't want to hear the negativity. Any variation or deviation would immediately result in the termination of my treatment. While desperately trying to help her, I was also attempting to protect myself from the pain of another leukemia-related tragedy.. But I made it clear that I do not treat leukemia or even the prevention of it. All I can do is to strengthen the body's organs, blood, cell tissue, immune system, and pray every day (which I do) that her disease never returns. I dramatically changed the little girl's diet (the parents changed their diet too), added a comprehensive array of living foods, provided an extensive pre-scription of powerful herbs, vitamins, and minerals that we periodically amend, plus the wild blue-green algae every single day. In the past five or so years that I have been treating this little girl (who is not so little any-more), all of the other children in the hospital on her cancer ward have since relapsed and died. Touch wood, my wee girl is alive and extremely well. She just completed her school exams. Algae, of course, is not the only answer. But frankly, I would not dream of taking her off it.

THE BASICS

Wild blue-green algae, scientifically referred to as *Aphanizomenon flos aqua* (AFA), are non-flowering water plants. They are unique in sharing characteristics not only with plants and animals, but also with bacteria.[134] Like plants, they perform photosynthesis, converting sunlight to chloro-phyll, but far more efficiently than any other plant. Thus, they are the most chlorophyll-rich organisms on Earth.[135] Like animals, they have soft digestible cell walls that our bodies can use as food; many plants have indigestible cellulose structures. And like bacteria, they have cells that lack a membrane-bound nucleus; other algae and plants have a nucleus and pigments confined within distinct membranes. This makes it especially easy for the body to absorb this algae.

Algae aren't newcomers on the nutrition scene. They were the initial form of life on Earth, and a rich source of food for the first 30,000 years of human existence. For thousands of years, Chinese herbalists used algae for vitamin and mineral deficiencies. Both the Aztecs in Mexico, and the Incas of South America, harvested and traded edible algae from their lakes. Fossil records indicate that the blue-greens are the most primitive of all algae, dating back over 4 billion years. They have excelled in the survival game. While other plants and animal species have become extinct, the blue-greens flourish largely because of their ability to adapt to change.[136] Whereas it might take humans a million years to develop genetic informa-tion to adapt to excess radiation, blue-green algae would adjust in a few months.[137] But the source of the algae is crucial. These algae must not be confused with the toxic algae *cyanobacteria* in British lakes, rivers, and ponds. According to scientists these blue-green algae from Klamath Lake in Oregon are completely safe, incapable of producing toxins.[138]

Absorption Rate

The real power of this algae is that it is so easily digested. "You are not what you eat, you are what you eat and absorb," as I always say. For instance, it's possible to ingest a beta-carotene supplement pill, but not absorb it. It could pass through your body—and straight out again, unabsorbed! You can eat the best diet in the world . . . but if your body fails to absorb, assimilate, metabolize, or digest, then little or no good is derived. Likewise with vitamin or mineral pills: if your biochemical absorption system doesn't function properly, you will not assimilate very much of these expensive nutrients. But these algae are fully assimilable. For your personal use, algae can be bought in most health food stores or natural food markets. They are available in powder, liquid, tablets, or capsules.

In my practice, I have corrected many nutrient deficiencies, especially mineral imbalance, through the regular use of wild blue-green algae. Algae have a greater than 90 percent assimilation rate. They are so biologically suited to the human digestive system, virtually all their nutrients are absorbed quickly and efficiently—*even if your absorption system isn't working properly*. These algae help you to absorb the nutrients from other foods as well. Dosages can span a wide range. Build up slowly over a six-week period from $1/4$ teaspoon to 2 teaspoons daily. Capsules—build up to six capsules daily; and for liquids, start out with 1 full dropper, building up to 2–4 daily. Various factors will influence dosage requirements: level of activity, degree of imbalances and deficiencies, weight, and general health. Correct dosage levels should result in more energy and fewer changes. In my practice, I often use the complementary blue-green algae *spirulina* together with the AFA blue-green. A dose of 1 heaping teaspoon (6 tablets) seems to be quite beneficial.

Nutritional Content and Benefits

While there are so many benefits to wild blue-green algae, the major reason that I include it in the "List of 12 Superfoods" is because of its overall harmonizing effect. First, it is harmonizing to the physiological and biological actions of the human body. Second, it harmonizes the other eleven superfoods I focus on in this book. The algae do not necessarily have super high potency of any one nutritional constituent, but they contain a fully balanced array of just about every known nutrient. Due to its molecular structure as a food, the absorption rate is unsurpassed. Let's look at this more closely.

This microorganism contains high-quality digestible vitamins, minerals, amino acids, and live enzymes. Its molecular structure consists of 60 percent protein, a more complete amino-acid profile than beef or soybeans, and it is the most potent food source of beta-carotene, vitamin B_{12}, and chlorophyll.

Vital Vitamins

The vitamin composition of blue-green algae is in perfect harmony and balance with human biochemistry for maximum utilization.[139] For example, these algae are rich in B vitamins, especially B_2, B_6, and B_{12}, essential for the production of red blood cells. The B vitamins transfer glucose into energy, and thus AFA algae might boost both your physical and mental stamina. The vitamin C composition in the algae helps the body to absorb the mineral iron.

Mighty Minerals

Not only are these algae rich in iron, but they have a full spectrum of minerals that are in perfect balance. I treat my patients with algae both to prevent and correct mineral deficiencies and imbalances. Minerals are the framework for our bodies, critical to our physical and mental health. They enable other nutrients to pass into the bloodstream; a deficiency in even one mineral can cause a host of vitamin imbalances and organ weaknesses.

Powerful Protein

Algae contain approximately 60 percent protein of a quality superior to that of other plants, since it's derived from all eight essential amino acids. Most plants lack certain amino acids; but if even one amino acid is missing, then the body cannot make protein. Meat usually contains all eight: but we absorb just about 20 percent of the protein in beef compared to approximately 85 percent in algae.[140]

Protein is vital for general health. In particular, the protein found in algae nourishes the brain and nervous system because of its high level of amino acid peptides (brain transmitters), which cross the blood-brain barrier. Studies have shown improved academic results when children take AFA algae.[141] And it may halt, reverse, or even prevent the progression of Alzheimer's disease according to laboratory tests.[142]

In his book *Beating Alzheimer's,* medical researcher Tom Warren claims to have cured himself and others of Alzheimer's disease. His research and biochemical tests are quite convincing. Warren's premise is that Alzheimer's disease sufferers do not have enough complete protein in the brain. When he corrects the protein imbalance, he also corrects the disease. For this reason, Warren prescribes algae for its comprehensive amino acid and complete protein profile.

The Importance of Enzymes

In blue-green algae, there are literally thousands of live active enzymes that help to improve digestive absorption so that the body can take up more immune-building anti-aging nutrients. The composition of the food we eat determines how much energy it takes to digest it. Blue-green algae require very little energy at all and are fully assimilated in about ninety seconds. But the more processed the food, the harder our bodies have to work, and the added strain we place on our army of enzymes struggling to digest it. Most people don't have enough enzymes. The body manufactures some, and the rest are acquired from foods.[143] Raw fruits and vegetables are packed with active enzymes, but they're easily destroyed through processing, cooking, or freezing. Algae deliver most active enzymes.

Pigments

Algae are rich in all kinds of botanical pigments—molecules capable of absorbing wavelengths of light and reflecting them as a recognizable color. It is my contention that these pigments have the ability to transmit essential metaphysical frequencies and invisible waves beneficial to human health, on a physical, emotional, and spiritual level. I'll mention just two and discuss their more physical attributes:

1. *Chlorophyll,* used to treat pain, ulcers, and skin disorders early in the twentieth century, was replaced by chemical antiseptics after World War II. Now there is renewed interest in this green plant substance, which can help regenerate damaged liver cells, increase circulation, and improve the heart's efficiency.[144] In my own practice, I have used chloro-

phyll to speed healing, prevent infection, act as an anti-inflammatory, and even combat bad breath and body odor. (See chlorophyll in the chapter on barley grass, page 66.)

2. *Beta-carotene* is a powerful antioxidant that boosts the immune system and protects against infection, allergies, and aging. The chlorophyll and enzymes in algae convert twice as much beta-carotene into vitamin A as other foods.[145] Twenty-five years of worldwide research shows that people who eat foods high in beta-carotene have less lung, stomach, colon, bladder, uterus, ovary, and skin cancers.[146]

CLINICAL USES

In my book *The Miracle Superfood: Wild Blue-Green Algae,* I present research on how algae stimulate immune response, improve digestion, detoxify the body, enhance tissue repair, accelerate healing, protect against radiation, help prevent degenerative diseases, and promote healthier life.

At my clinic, I have found it successful in treating:

1. *Candida albicans*—it essentially dries the excess fluids and helps drain "dampness" in which candida flourishes.[147]

2. *Depression*—it is high in the B vitamins, most often deficient in depressed people.

3. *Liver fatigue*—it contains an amino acid capable of detoxifying harmful compounds in the liver. It also provides the liver with assimilable protein to help fight infection.

4. *Heavy metal poisoning*—it stimulates the discharge of toxic residues, builds up the blood, and renews cellular tissue.

5. *Weight loss and sweet cravings*—it calms blood sugar fluctuations and keeps the appetite under control.

6. *Anti-aging*—the antioxidant beta-carotene helps protect against premature aging, and the rich enzyme content helps absorption of anti-aging nutrients.

7. *Anemia*—it is rich in iron, folic acid, vitamin B_{12}, and vitamin E, which build blood.

8. *Skin conditions*—beta-carotene, which is converted to vitamin A, is

beneficial for skin eruptions, healing damaged tissue, and constructing new skin.

9. *Poor memory and lack of concentration*—its protein and large number of neuropeptides (brain transmitters) nourish the brain, improving mental clarity.

Bowel Mover

Miss T, a well-known television actress, was totally blocked when she first came to see me. She had never moved her bowels regularly, suffering from constipation since childhood. She sometimes did not move her bowels for up to six days! She also suffered from fluid retention in her ankles. Stool tests revealed a major imbalance of gut flora and some pathogenic bacteria. Blood results revealed low magnesium, folic acid, and iron, which also can contribute to poor elimination and constipation. Her tongue often appeared sore, with a dark-red coloring and thick coating. This suggested to me that her liver was stagnant with reduced energy flow through the gastrointestinal areas. Her bowel movements were usually dry and hard, indicating a "hot" or "inflamed" liver; liver inflammation is frequently the result of poor diet exacerbated by poor elimination. This type of liver stagnancy reduces peristalsis, the wavelike muscular contraction of the intestines. Result: delayed bowel movements. Algae may be the best remedy for combating liver degradation or imbalances. AFA algae are one of the few blue-green algae that contain chlorine; a deficiency of chlorine can cause fatty degeneration of the liver, venous congestion, and constipation.

Everyone is at risk of liver fatigue, the swelling or sluggishness of this important organ. Studies now show that poor diet, stressful lifestyle, medications, and alcohol and environmental pollutants cause untold damage and degradation to our livers.[148] Some symptoms of liver fatigue are constipation, indigestion, skin disorder, swollen glands, a feeling of a lump in your throat, menstrual problems, depression, and bodily pains. Your liver needs to be able to process and destroy harmful substances such as drugs, poisons, chemicals, viruses, and bacterial infections. The liver stores important nutrients, produces others, and recreates a fluid called bile for digestion.

I started Miss T on a gentle program of blue-green algae.

Week 1:   ¾ teaspoon blue-green algae

Week 2:   ½ teaspoon   mixed with
                                                   aloe vera juice
Week 3:   ¾ teaspoon   in apple juice

Week 4:   1 teaspoon

First, wild blue-green algae have a very mild diuretic action, thus reducing the fluid retention in Miss T. Second, wild blue-green algae have a "cooling" effect on the body. It won't make you cold, but it encourages the body to contract, pushing the energy lower down. The wild blue-green algae will consequently "cool" the heat in the liver. Third, the bitter action of the wild blue-green algae enters the intestines and increases muscle contractions and peristalsis. Result: more efficient bowel movements. Miss T now moves her bowels every day, usually twice daily. Miss T's mineral levels and gut flora have normalized. She reports an abundant increase of mental energy, too.

Proper bowel elimination rids the body of toxins and bacteria, ultimately helping you to feel well. The average healthy person ought to move the bowels two to three times each day. In fact, new research suggest that infrequent or incomplete bowel elimination may result in an array of ailments including diabetes mellitus, meningitis, myasthenia gravis, thyroid disease, diverticulitis, and ulcerative colitis, just to name a few.

Case Study: Dorothy, 35, Patient

Since age seventeen, after a bout of glandular fever, Dorothy had continual fingernail problems: the nails had been brittle, covered in white spots and chipped easily. This condition is known as leukonykia, and is often linked with a zinc deficiency and malabsorption. By thirty-five years of age, Dorothy had arrived at my clinic complaining that the nail problem had accelerated and was now accompanied by excessive hair loss.

Blood tests and hair mineral analysis revealed low levels of vitamin B_{12}, folate, and zinc. Over the years, Dorothy had tried all types of nutrients including multimineral complexes, the B vitamins, and four different types of zinc (liquid, capsule, tablet, and lozenge).

Dorothy was amazed to find out through my blood tests and hair analysis that she was still zinc deficient after all these years of supplementation. She simply was not absorbing zinc and other nutrients and minerals. Zinc absorption may vary from about 20 to 40 percent of ingested zinc.

Dorothy's Algae Program

Weeks 1 and 2: $\frac{1}{2}$ teaspoon daily ($\frac{1}{2}$ gram)

Weeks 3 and 4: 1 teaspoon daily (1 gram)

Weeks 5–8: 2 teaspoons daily (2 grams)

Weeks 9–12: 2 heaped teaspoons daily (4 grams)

Weeks 13–16: 2 heaped teaspoons twice daily (8 grams)

Weeks 17–21: decreased dosage to 2 teaspoons daily (4 grams)

To follow, a maintenance program of 1 teaspoon per day (1 gram).

After six weeks on my program of algae, Dorothy's white spots on the fingernails had started to diminish. After sixteen weeks, the white spots had disappeared completely; the hair was no longer falling out. The patient also claims to have more energy and recently became pregnant after four years of failed attempts.

Comments on Dorothy

Although Dorothy was ingesting different forms of zinc for years, she was obviously not absorbing this important mineral. Deficiency of zinc is associated with the maintenance of body tissues, sexual function, reproductive system, immunity, and detoxification. Research now shows that zinc is probably involved in more body functions than any other mineral. Although the dosages of the various nutrients in the algae are relatively low, the absorption rate and the body's ability to metabolize the blue-green algae are outstanding.

WORLDWIDE RESEARCH

Blue-green algae are currently used throughout the world with great success.[149]

- Scientists at the U.S. Cancer Research Institute have found that chemicals derived from blue-green algae inhibit the growth of the AIDS virus.[150]

- NASA has been testing various algae as a food source for astronauts.[151] Their findings were published in *The Journal of the National Cancer Institute*.[152]

- The Russians used blue-green algae to treat patients exposed to radiation in the Chernobyl disaster.

- The Kanembus tribe still eat algae from Lake Chad in Africa, and their children don't suffer from malnutrition, unlike their non-algae eating neighbors.

- The Japanese use blue-green algae to heal wounds, particularly gangrenous feet.

- And in 1994, a study in Nicaragua proved that just 1 gram of AFA algae a day, for six months, returned malnourished school children to good health.

IN A NUTSHELL

In a nutshell, wild blue-green algae is a superb natural food source of nutrients for the body. I see algae as a harmonizer of energy compounds. It boasts outstanding levels of chlorophyll, beta-carotene, iron, protein, and many more complementary nutrients in a completely assimilable form. As a result, the wild blue-green algae can help to increase energy, correct imbalances, oxygenate cells, and help us to realize high levels of physical and mental health.

As a "bitter" substance, it influences the heart and mind, helping to clean out damp accumulations from the arteries, thus stabilizing blood pressure. The bitterness can also help to focus the mind and improve concentration. As a "drying" substance, algae can remove excessive mucosal moisture from tissues, rendering these cells a less favorable environment for viruses, bacteria, parasites, and fungi. Yeasts, tumor or cyst growths, excess phlegm, abscesses, swellings, edema, and skin eruptions all might respond well to algae. It has also been used for patients suffering from cancer, AIDS, Epstein-Barr, MS, and rheumatoid arthritis where internal

"wet conditions" exist. The algae also acts as a "coolant," thus aiding constipation, inflammations, infections, and fevers. The algae make amino acids
readily available to the brain, thereby stimulating neurotransmitters for
improved mental acuity and memory. Finally, AFA algae is a relaxant. Its
predigested proteins and complex carbohydrates maintain balanced blood
sugar levels, supplying energy that lasts.

Wild blue-green algae can benefit almost everyone. If you have
grown up on meat and potatoes, eggs, dairy products, salty foods, chemically preserved foods, and sugary foods, then algae is for you. If you eat
on the run, need to lose weight, feel tired, have poor nutritional habits,
then this algae is also for you. Even if you think you are the most healthy
of specimens, I still recommend the algae. It is a complete source of
wholesome nutrients in a world where our foods are so nutrient-deplet-
ed. It rejuvenates your lungs, purifies the kidneys, feeds the gastrointestinal tract, and nurtures the brain as it harmonizes and balances all
meridians. Wild blue-green algae is a true builder of your body, an amazing cleaner and blood purifier. Wild blue-green algae may be more
bioavailable than virtually all other natural food sources or food supplements. This means that the algae, because of its delicate balance, can
assimilate, absorb, digest, and metabolize in perfect harmony for maximum beneficial results.

HOW TO TAKE BLUE-GREEN ALGAE
Dosages
Your initial introduction to wild blue-green algae should begin slowly.
This potent micro-algae food is new to your body; your system may need
time to adjust to its effects. It is best to start with the minimum dosage and
increase it according to your needs. You may need to do some experimenting, or better yet, consult a qualified nutritionist or informed health
practitioner. Various factors will influence dosage requirements: level of
activity, degree of imbalances and deficiencies, weight, and general health.
The correct dosage level should result in more energy and fewer cravings.
Some may notice an increase in physical and mental energy quite early in
the program. Correct dosages can span a wide range. I have patients on
dosages ranging from 2–10 grams daily, depending upon personal symptoms and specific biochemical needs.

In very general terms, I recommend gradually working up to approximately two good size teaspoons every day for the best, long-term results. But everyone's biochemistry is so different. Listen to your body as some may need higher dosages for best results; some may require lower dosages. Small amounts can still make a big difference in the way you feel.

The more "unbalanced" or toxic the person is, the less micro-algae should be taken at the beginning. For rejuvenating or detoxifying the liver, or for decreasing other major symptoms, plan on taking wild blue-green algae for at least a year. You may notice an increase in physical and mental energy quite early in an algae ingestion program. If you do not feel any difference in your health, you may be taking too little or you may already be at optimum health. Stress can cause a depletion of important nutrients in the body. During stressful times, you may need more algae (4–10 grams daily). Taking the algae at different times of the day can be a helpful boost.

Some people taking the algae for the first time may experience an adverse reaction, for example, a mild frontal headache or possibly diarrhea; it usually indicates a beneficial healing reaction, although in some cases, too much is being taken. The headache or diarrhea may be due to an adjustment of glucose metabolism. Eating complex carbohydrates should relieve the symptom. In either case, take less for a couple of weeks. Gradually increase the dosage again. Although it is preferable to take algae on an empty stomach or before meals, eating algae after meals or at mealtimes can often reduce any unpleasant reactions when introducing this new food into your diet.

Complementary Nutrients

In my practice, I often use the complementary blue-green algae spirulina together with the AFA blue-green algae. A heaping teaspoon of spirulina (6 tablets) seems to be quite beneficial. I also suggest to my clients that they take an enzyme supplement with each meal of the day to help with absorption of nutrients from the algae and other foods.

With chronic arthritis, take small dosages in the beginning. Increase gradually, as micro-algae may initially increase pain as toxins are moved out of the system. Similarly, if you suffer chronic intestinal symptoms, you may actually experience additional flatulence at the outset of the program.

Micro-algae may initially increase fermentation in the gut as it destroys noxious bacteria. This flatulence will subside. (Special note for men only: an algae regimen may enhance sperm count, potency, and endurance.) Algae can often have a strong cleansing and detoxification action when first introduced to your system. Therefore, I recommend a slow buildup as follows:

Powders:

Mix powders in large glass of water or juice	Week 1:	$\frac{1}{4}$ tsp daily	1 tsp = approx. 1 gram
	Week 2:	$\frac{1}{2}$ tsp daily	
	Week 3:	$\frac{3}{4}$ tsp daily	
	Week 4:	1 tsp daily	
	Week 5:	$1\frac{1}{2}$ tsp daily	
	Week 6:	2 tsp daily	

Capsules or tablets:

Tablets could be chewed for best absorption and results.

Drink 1 large glass of water after taking tablets or capsules.	Week 1:	1 daily	4 capsules = approx. 1 gram
	Week 2:	2 daily	
	Week 3:	3 daily	
	Week 4:	4 daily	

Liquid:

Mix drops in large glass of water or juice	Week 1:	1 full dropper	Standard dosage = 2–4 full droppers
	Week 2:	2 full droppers	
	Week 3:	3 full droppers	
	Week 4:	4 full droppers	

Remember, however, that these are very general recommendations as a basic guideline only; each person's biochemistry, deficiencies, imbalances and lifestyle is so different and may require completely different dosages.

DR. GILLIAN'S ALGAE AVOCADO CREAM SAUCE

4 tbsp water (preferably still mineral water)

2 very ripe avocados

2 stalks of finely chopped fresh raw spring onions

¼ tsp of coriander powder

¼ tsp of salt

½ tsp olive oil

½ level teaspoon algae powder

Place the water (approximately 4 tbsp) in a blender.

Then add raw avocados, spring onion, coriander, salt, olive oil, and algae powder into the blender, and mix until all smooth and creamy.

The consistency should be a fluffy soft cream. Use this cream as a delicious topping for salmon.

The avocado cream sauce may also be used as a dressing for salad.

Note: Avocados contain 14 minerals to regulate body functions. They are high in lecithin, which feeds the brain and reduces fat in the body. They are an excellent source of protein and prevent anemia.

Spring onions remove heavy metals.

Coriander powder has twice as much vitamin C as oranges.

DR. GILLIAN MCKEITH'S ALGAE ENERGIZER

4-6 organic carrots

1 stalk celery

¼ inch fresh ginger root

sprig of fresh parsley

1 dropper of liquid algae;
or ½ level teaspoon of algae powder

Process all the ingredients through the juicer and enjoy. Great for boosting flagging energy levels.

If you find vegetable juices heavy going at first, add the juice of ½ to 1 apple. The apple juice will lighten up the flavor.

ALGAE SELF-TEST

Is this you?

If you answer "yes" to one or more of the following symptoms, you may benefit from including algae in your daily regimen:

❏ Malabsorption

❏ Nutrient deficiencies

❏ Poor digestion

❏ Constipation

❏ Lack of concentration

❏ Run-down feeling

❏ Lack of energy

❏ Liver problems

❏ White spots on nails

❏ Infections/colds

❏ Poor memory

❏ Depression

❏ Mucus congestion

❏ Yeast problems

If you exhibit one to three of the above symptoms, you may need algae two to three times weekly.

If you exhibit four to ten of the above symptoms, you may need algae every other day.

If you exhibit eleven to fourteen of the above symptoms, you may need algae on a daily basis over the short term. (If you have a "cold" constitution, that is, feel cold a lot, make sure you include plenty of warming herbs in your diet.) Please read the section on dosage levels.

14.

THE RAW RESEARCH

The Case Against Cooking

The living foods are packed with enzymes; that is their primary benefit. The greatest threat to our food enzymes is the very act of cooking (boiling, baking, frying, etc.); all cooked foods are devoid of all enzymes. When any food is heated above 118°F for approximately 20 minutes, there is complete and total devastation of all enzymes within that specific food.[153] My point is clearly illustrated by the acclaimed Pottenger Study under the personal direction of Francis Pottenger, M.D., and reported in the *American Journal of Orthodontics and Oral Surgery*.[154] A ten-year, four-generation study of 900 cats was conducted, and half of the cats were fed raw meat and milk; the remaining half of the cats were fed cooked meats and pasteurized (heat-processed) milk.

The cats eating the cooked foods developed a litany of degenerative diseases, not unlike the illnesses in modern Western society. In fact, each generation of these cats dramatically deteriorated with congenital bone problems, osteoporosis and arthritic disorders, immune dysfunction, and even sterility, and congenital deformation and birth defects by the third and fourth generations. The cats on raw meats and unpasteurized milk did not suffer this ill fate. The Pottenger Study concludes that it was the absolute absence of enzymes that caused these abnormalities and degenerative diseases. (This study is not to be construed as advocacy for humans eating raw meats. I would never advocate anyone to eat *raw* meats. The study is meant only to illustrate the importance of *enzymes*.)

Lost Protein

Cooking not only destroys enzymes, but protein is not spared either by heat. When we cook high-protein foods too vigorously, the protein itself is actually destroyed, rendered at least useless, or at worst harmful. For example, a study reported in the *Journal of Nutrition Review* stated that the amino acid lysine (a protein constituent) was found to be indigestible and unable to be assimilated with other amino acids for protein formation.[155] Another study on protein loss in cooked meat, sponsored by the U.S. Department of Agriculture, concluded that "cooking at 400°F (the average temperature for cooking meats), caused a very marked decrease (four- to thirty-fold) in the soluble protein of the steaks under analysis."[156] While so many people are fixated on getting their protein from meats, the fact is that they are probably obtaining little or no usable protein from their cooked meats anyway, due to the high cooking temperature.

Destruction of Vitamins

As if that were not enough, we now move on to the destruction of vitamins in cooking. Not only does cooking destroy all the enzymes, but it degrades most of the vitamin activity too. Although not all vitamins are destroyed from high heat, the vitamin activity is enormously curtailed. It is estimated that no less than 50 percent of B vitamins are lost through cooking. Some of the individual B vitamins are drastically reduced even further. For instance, the loss of thiamine (B_1) can be as high as a 96 percent reduction if the food is boiled for a prolonged period of time. Similarly, up to 72 percent of biotin can be lost, up to 97 percent of folic acid lost, up to 95 percent of inositol lost, and up to 80 percent of vitamin C lost, all from cooking. In fact, according to one of the world's leading researchers on the topic, Dr. Viktoras Kulvinskas, in his *Survival Report Into The 21st Century,* cooking will cause an average overall nutrient loss of up to 85 percent.[157] This means that we are often only obtaining less than 15 percent of the nutritive value of most foods, a lesser percentage of protein, and too frequently zero percent of the enzymes in these same foods.

Other Problems

Finally, eating overly hot foods is certainly not doing any favors for our bodily functions either, causing other enzymatic problems. My own father-in-law insists on drinking his tea so hot that it would scald any other mortal's mouth. A study published in the *Lancet* medical journal reported that

15 percent of people who drank tea above 122°F, and 77 percent of those who drank tea above 137°F, had "gastric enzymatic abnormalities."[158] In other words, digestion becomes impaired when you drink beverages or eat foods that are simply too hot. In another study reported in the *Lancet,* researcher Dr. C. McCluskey found that constantly eating overly hot food irritates the molecular cell structure of the mouth and tongue, ultimately increasing the risk of tongue and throat cancers.[159]

Perhaps the most shocking assertion is that a diet full of cooked foods causes the reduction of brain tissue and the swelling of the key organs! The eminent Edward Howell, M.D., who spent a lifetime researching enzyme biochemistry, wrote volumes on the results of laboratory animals. When rats were fed diets devoid of enzymes (that is, cooked or canned foods only) their brains actually shrank. In addition, serious other disturbances occurred with the experimental animals: the endocrine system, pituitary, thyroid, pancreas, kidneys, liver, heart, spleen, and other organs swelled. Swollen organs mean weakened organs, ultimately malfunctioning or non-functioning organs, a rather grave prospect. Howell cites more than 50 prominent studies from around the world to support his claims, including the *Harvard Medical School Study* by Doctors N. B. Marshall, S. B. Andrus and J. Mayer, whereby they found that the organs of mice grotesquely enlarged.[160]

Moreover, during cooking, agricultural pesticides and fungicides could release into the foods to form even more toxic compounds.[161] These poisons settle in weak areas of the body, further burdening the liver; expelling them is difficult. Whenever possible, do your best to buy organic produce to avoid or at least lessen this problem. Organic produce should be free of adverse bacteria, pesticides, herbicides, insecticides, fungicides, dioxins, and more byproducts of destructive agricultural practices.

Immune Collapse

Too-vigorous cooking not only causes organ and cell tissue abnormalities, but ultimately compromises the overall immune system. Cooked foods have shown to adversely alter blood structure, thus weakening immune response. A research paper was presented by Paul Kouchakoff, M.D., at the first International Congress of Microbiology titled "The Influence of Cooking Food on the Blood Formula of Man."[162] This paper reported that eating cooked food caused a medical condition referred to as leukocytosis, and is extremely weakening to the immune system. Interestingly enough, even just a small amount of cooked food could cause leukocytosis. Leukocytosis, the abnormal increase of the white blood cells, is like the body constantly fighting an infection. When we get ill, the white blood cells increase in order to combat the illness. But with leukocytosis, caused by eating only cooked foods, it is as though our defense system is on continual high alert. Such a state ultimately leads to other physiological and biochemical changes as well. If I may indulge in some hypothesizing and some logical assumptions as a nutritional biochemist, I must next pose the potentiality that a perpetual state of high alert could easily lead to full collapse of the immune function.

Combat Fatigue

In effect, if the white blood cells are constantly elevated due to a poor diet of only cooked foods, then the immune system may be unable to recognize a real bacterial or viral invader. In other words, because the white blood cells are constantly having to overwork, overproduce, and overexert, they can no longer perform properly when a real infection sets in. I always say that fighting illness is just like going to war. But a good general would never keep his infantry on full military alert all the time. Eventually, the troops are changed, rotated, removed, or the high alert is downgraded so that the soldiers are kept fresh, renewed, regenerated. In military terms, they call this preventing "battle fatigue." The same holds true with our blood cells. Keep the white blood cells on high alert all the time, and they run the risk of combat fatigue. Give the white blood cells a rest from high alert and they can be more responsive, more receptive, fresher. Similarly, imagine constantly revving your car engine; eventually it becomes flooded, and it cannot work properly. In a sense, an all-cooked foods diet "floods" the blood system, the immune system, and the organs. The end result is that you get sick more frequently, or you simply just feel tired, or worse.

RAW BALANCES THE COOKED

The exciting news here, however, is that the presenting researcher at that International Congress of Microbiology, Paul Kouchakoff, M.D., emphatically pointed out that eating raw foods, or even just foods heated below 190°F, could prevent any rise in white blood cells. Perhaps most significantly, though, was that Dr. Kouchakoff found that eating an approximate 50–50 ratio of raw foods to cooked foods could also prevent leukocytosis.

For this reason, I advise my own patients that when you eat cooked foods also have some raw or low-heated food at the same meal. Thus, try to eat raw foods with cooked foods at the same time to avert the destructive impact upon blood cells. Cooked foods need only to be simmered or steamed lightly. Therefore, I find the Kouchakoff Study actually rather liberating, because it provides enough information to allow you the best of both worlds. You can still eat cooked foods, but just balance it with more raw.

Climatic and Bodily Adaptation

So you will not be shocked to learn that I do not advocate an all-raw foods diet. Maybe if you live in a warm, sunny, dry climate, all year, a diet of raw fresh fruits and raw vegetables with raw sprouts sounds perfect. But from my own clinical experience, I can assure you that eating all-raw simply does not work for the majority of the population in modern Western society. I have had certain patients come to me who were rather lethargic after embarking upon such a raw regime. A few of these patients had arrived with weakened organs, fatigue, and immune dysfunction. The all-raw diet was simply too taxing on the liver, spleen, and kidneys for these cold-climate people.

I'll give you an example close to home. My own mother-in-law once went to an all-raw cleansing center where she ate raw foods for three weeks. She would be the first to tell you that her stay there did true wonders for her health. Many ailments completely disappeared after the three weeks on the raw regimen. But this seventy-year-old woman normally lives in the seasonally defined climate of the American Northeast— Philadelphia: severely frozen in the winter, often rather wet and damp in the spring or autumn. Suddenly, she is whisked to sunny, hot, dry California, embarking upon an all-raw foods diet plus colonics—a colonic is like an enema, but forty times more powerful.

On the sixth day in California, she actually collapsed in her hotel room. The differentials were too great: different climate, different foods, too much bowel movement, and so on. But the greatest deficit was the lack of support to the organs. The organs require a certain amount of "warm" and warming foods for balance. One of the biggest problems with trying to eat an all-raw diet in climates where there is a change of weather, or especially cold weather, is that there is no way that people—especially those from northern counties—can feel completely well on this diet. When the climate is cold, even just a tad chilly, it is the normal inclination for our species to seek out warmer foods. And that is the operative word: warm.

My Secret

Therefore, I recommend that when you are cooking fruit and vegetables, it is better to warm them whenever possible rather than vigorously cook them. For example, in the cold months, I make a delicious split pea soup for my family, which everyone loves (you will find the recipe in Chapter 9). It does indeed require some cooking to create the soup. But I still manage to get in the raw. Here's what I do. Once the soup is hot and ready to serve, I then add various fresh raw vegetables just moments before it hits the table. I might add raw snow peas, raw chopped carrot, or even raw diced broccoli to the completed soup. Thus, the soup may have gone through the cooking process, but the added fresh raw vegetables were only warmed by the soup broth. Thus, the family enjoys warm soup in the winter, while I enjoy knowing they're all getting a substantial ration of raw vegetables in the soup.

I do much the same in autumn and spring with my famous Dreamy Creamy Fruit Smoothie (famous only to my family). Here's where I might take some fresh seasonal fruits like pears and apples, simmer them briefly, and then blend to a creamy consistency. Add some fresh raw strawberries or other seasonal berries to the apple and pear cream. The apples and pears may have been lightly cooked in order to soften them, but the berries were added at the end completely raw. If my husband gets his way, he might wildly throw in some raw mint leaves. Then blend again. I even then add my Living Food Energy Powder into the creamy mix, and blend one last time. The end result is that we get to eat this *warm* dreamy fruit pudding on cold mornings, with some raw foods mixed in. We all feel satisfied. I must confess, however, we do consume a lot of fruit using this method, especially whatever is fresh and in season. For a while, my husband used to call me the "Mango Queen" (see my Mango Mania recipe on page 140). That's all changed—he now calls me "The Papaya Princess"! (see my recipe for Papaya Heaven on page 140).

To conclude today's lesson, I hope it is now clear that I am not saying you should never eat cooked foods again. In fact, I am saying quite the contrary: I want you to include *more* raw live foods in your daily diet, *less* cooked. During cold winter or rainy months, I would certainly urge the inclusion of some warm foods. There are also those foods that are "warming" foods. For example, cinnamon, garlic, quinoa sprouts, and ginger are foods that "warm" the body, whether served raw, cold, or warm. (See chart of Warming Foods below.) These foods serve an important function in our bodies, helping to circulate the blood and comfort the organs. "Warming" foods may not necessarily be served warm, but they do indeed help to warm the body.

So now you know my secret. I prepare many different cooked soups, casseroles, and stews in winter. Then I might add specific raw vegetables or fresh raw seasonings at the very end. So, in effect, the vegetables are only warmed by the main dish, though not necessarily cooked. These added vegetables only need to be heated for just the last two minutes, or even just the last thirty seconds for that matter, thus maintaining most of the benefits of the "rawness." Nevertheless, the bottom line is that raw live foods and sprouts provide us with a broader range of active nutrients and enzymes than any other way of eating.

Warming Herbs/Seasonings

Basil	Cinnamon	Fennel	Mustard
Bay leaves	Cloves	Fenugreek	Nutmeg
Caraway	Coriander	Garlic	Oregano
Cardamom	Cumin	Ginger	Pepper
Chives	Dill	Lemongrass	Spearmint

Warming Sprouts

Fenugreek sprouts	Radish sprouts

DR. GILLIAN'S CREAMY BROCCOLI SOUP

3 heads broccoli

*6 cups water or more
(enough to cover vegetables)*

1 whole fennel, diced

1 vegetable bouillon cube

handful fresh tarragon

¼ cup fresh sage leaves

1 cup fresh sprouts

Add cut broccoli to hot water. Simmer for 7 minutes. Turn off heat and add all other ingredients *except* sprouts.

Blend in a food processor. You may adjust soup consistency by adding more or less water.

Add sprouts into blender at the end, or serve soup with whole sprouts as a garnish.

A variation to this recipe is to add different herbs such as fresh parsley, cilantro, or dill.

DR. GILLIAN McKEITH'S MANGO MANIA

2 soft ripe mango fruits

1 soft ripe peach

1 banana

Lemon juice (optional)

Blend all the ingredients until smooth and creamy—add a dash of lemon juice if you like.

PAPAYA PRINCESS

1 ripe papaya, peeled and deseeded

3 soft pears

6 strawberries

Blend all the ingredients until smooth and creamy.

Dr. Gillian's Winter Warmer

4 apples

2 pears

1 banana (optional)

6 strawberries

Peel the apples and pears and cut them in quarters. Gently simmer the fruit for 2-3 minutes, and strain off the liquid. Transfer the fruit to a blender, with the banana, if using and blend until smooth and creamy.

Serve garnished with chopped raw strawberries.

Fantastic!

15.

THE PATH TO PERFECT HEALTH

More Superfoods

You are now well aware of the twelve most important balanced and harmonized "living foods for energy" that strengthened me and ultimately my patients at the clinic. However, these living foods are not the entirety of all healthy live foods. There are many other sprouts, seeds, beans, nuts, grains, algae, and sea vegetables that I have not mentioned. But the specific foods that I highlight in this book are the ones with which I have had the most clinical success. They are also the ones that are most beneficial in harmonizing and neutralizing the effects of our modern Western diets and lifestyle.

For example, modern Western processed foods will often lead to weak spleens. My "list of 12" calls for generous amounts of millet sprouts, a toning agent for the spleen. Yet there are many other sprouted grains besides millet that may be beneficial for your health: for example oats, rice, amaranth, and spelt, to name just a few.

I have, therefore, prepared a compilation of additional living foods or superfoods not necessarily part of my prescription, but nonetheless beneficial for you to know about.

Grains

Grains are your basic energy food. They are largely composed of complex carbohydrates. When consumed, they are broken down slowly in the digestive system, creating glucose energy, and released into the blood as fuel. For this reason, complex carbohydrates are often referred to as the "building blocks for energy." Thus, virtually all unrefined grains can be beneficial to health. Processed grains, such as white rice, white bread, and white pasta, do not have the same beneficial actions. In fact, besides being robbed of all their nutrients and fiber (the majority of vitamins and minerals are found in the bran and germ, which are removed in the refining process), these processed grains behave more like sugar when ingested: rushing into the system and creating havoc. The outcome might be blood glucose disturbances, sugar cravings, and mood swings, as well as weight gain. That's why I recommend unrefined brown rice and the unrefined versions of grains like wheat berries, barley groats, and so on.

Nutrition and Beyond

Not only are unrefined grains an excellent source of complex carbohydrates, but they are a vital source of fiber, vitamin B complex and E, and a variety of minerals including calcium, magnesium, potassium, iron, zinc, copper, and selenium.

Protein-wise, grains have a lot to offer too. But because most of them do not contain all eight essential amino acids (protein building blocks), they need to be combined with complementary protein sources to make a complete protein; examples of these sources are beans, seeds, and pulses. This combining ritual doesn't have to be achieved in the same meal. As long as a variety of grains, beans, seeds, or pulses are eaten throughout the day, your needs should be adequately met. (Note: the grain quinoa, as recommended in my living food prescription, actually contains a superior *complete* protein—more usable protein than in meat!)

According to Eastern tenets, there's far more to grains than good nutrition. The cereal family is considered the most harmonizing, balancing, and stabilizing of foods.

Gluten

Some grains contain a substance called gluten. Gluten is a sticky protein-carbohydrate component found typically in wheat, rye, and oats. Due to the overconsumption of wheat in the West, many individuals have developed an intolerance to it. Symptoms of gluten sensitivity include bloating, abdominal pain, diarrhea, anemia, depression, and weight loss. If you think that gluten may be causing you a problem, switch to the gluten-free grains (millet, quinoa, buckwheat, rice, and amaranth), and see if your symptoms subside.

Eating Guidelines

• Eat only those grains that are unrefined, not processed.

- Wash grains well before cooking. Cook until soft and all the water has been absorbed (see grain cooking chart).

- Chew them well. This will improve digestion.

- Try sprouting your favorite grains as frequently as possible. Did you know the gluten content of wheat virtually disappears once germinated as sprouts?

- Store grains in sealed containers and use within four months of purchasing. I normally keep my own grains in the fridge or freezer (especially during warm summer months).

GRAIN COOKING CHART			
Grain	Amount of Grain in Cups	Amount of Water in Cups	Cooking Time
Amaranth	1	$2\frac{1}{2}$	35 mins
Pot Barley*	1	3	1 hour
Buckwheat (roasted)	1	2	20 mins
Millet	1	3	45 mins
Oat groats (whole)*	1	2	1 hour
Quinoa	1	2	15 mins
Brown Rice	1	2	35 mins

*Soak overnight

My Super Eight List

After quinoa and millet, the following grains are excellent living foods.

1. Brown Rice

As a rich source of B vitamins, rice is beneficial for the nervous system. Eaten regularly, rice may help relieve the symptoms of depression.[163] Rice compounds and "energies" are particularly beneficial to the stomach and spleen, and are helpful for diarrhea and thirst. The short grain variety is particularly good for colon function, helping to clear toxic waste.

Short grain: Eat in autumn and winter

Long grain: Eat in summer

Basmati rice: Perfect for people who are overweight or internally "mucousy."

2. Barley

Barley is probably the oldest of cultivated cereals. The pearl variety is the name given to the refined form; pot barley is the whole grain. Barley has a sweet flavor, is good for digestion as its energies help to strengthen the tummy and spleen. It is helpful in cases of edema, indigestion, and dryness. Barley does contain gluten, although gluten quantities are low. Do not confuse barley with barley grass. They are completely different foods. Barley grass does *not* contain gluten, a substance to which some people may be sensitive.

3. Oats

Oats are high in protein and contain more "good" fat than other grains. It is a rich source of vitamin B, and therefore is beneficial to the nervous system. Oats strengthen bones and connective tissue; they contain high amounts of silicon.[164] They are available in several forms: whole, jumbo, and the finer rolled and meal. Oats are "warming" to the body. As they are mucus forming, avoid if you suffer from excess phlegm, catarrh, or sinusitis. Besides eating them for breakfast, add them to soups, toppings, and desserts.

4. Buckwheat

Buckwheat is gluten-free and therefore beneficial for people who are sensitive to high-gluten grains like wheat. It contains about 15 to 20 percent protein and the bioflavonoid rutin, which strengthens blood capillaries and assists the circulatory system. This makes it a good food for the prevention and treatment of varicose veins. Buckwheat combines nicely with vegetables for delicious savories and salads. Cook with ginger or "warming" herbs if you feel the cold; as buckwheat has a "cooling" effect on the body. It is toning to the blood, stomach, spleen, and colon.

5. Amaranth

This ancient grain served as a staple for the Aztecs of Central America more than 6,000 years ago. Around the 1500s, it was banished as a crop by invaders, but has recently made a comeback. Like quinoa, amaranth too is a complete protein. Because it has a high lysine content (most grains lack this amino acid), when mixed with other grains, a superior protein is formed. This makes it particularly good for people who need more protein. Finally, amaranth is one of the richest vegetable sources of iron. It is beneficial for those with yeast problems, as it helps to dry up excess-mucus conditions.

6. Spelt

Spelt is from the same genus as modern wheat, with a similar look and taste. However, due to the solubility of its gluten content, spelt is a better option. It also possesses 30 percent more protein than wheat, and does not seem to create allergic reactions like wheat. Spelt is the only grain containing mucopolysaccharides. According to the *Journal of Medical Plant Research,* these mucopolysaccharides from spelt assist blood clotting and stimulate the immune system.[165] Colitis, poor digestion, and constipation are conditions that will benefit.

7. Teff

Teff is a flavorful tiny seed. It is five times higher in iron, calcium, and potassium than most other grains. It contains substantial amounts of protein and fiber.

8. Kamut

Kamut is an ancient grain closely related to wheat. However, many allergic people who react to wheat seem to tolerate kamut. Some researchers have hypothesized that this is because the kamut has not been genetically hybridized. Nutritionally, kamut has about twice as much protein as wheat. It contains more minerals than wheat, especially magnesium and zinc. Kamut has sixteen amino acids and essential fatty acids too.

Organ Strengthening Chart

Grains	Organs
Amaranth	Lungs
Barley	Spleen/pancreas
Buckwheat	Intestine
Corn	Heart
Millet	Stomach, spleen, liver
Oats	Spleen/pancreas
Quinoa	Kidneys/whole body
Rice	Spleen/pancreas
Spelt	Spleen/pancreas
Wheat*	Heart/mind/kidneys

Most of us eat far too much wheat. Overuse of wheat can ultimately exert a negative effect on the blood and organs.

Beans

Known collectively as legumes, sometimes referred to as pulses, beans are basically seeds from a pod of a specific group of plants. Ideally, they should form part of your daily diet. Legumes are packed with protein; however, they need to be combined with grains for the protein to be complete. The soybean is the exception, as it contains all eight essential amino acids. Legumes also possess a supply of carbohydrates, vitamins, and minerals, including B vitamins, calcium, magnesium, potassium, zinc, iron, and phosphorus. Legumes are carriers of the two essential types of fiber, soluble and insoluble. These fibers work together in reducing cholesterol levels and maintaining colon regularity.

Preparation Tips

For maximum digestibility of beans, follow these tips:

- With the exception of red lentils, soak all dry beans for at least three hours or even overnight in plenty of water. Then drain and rinse.

- For quickness, choose to pressure cook larger legumes, rather than boil.

- Whatever softening method you opt for, feel free to add a few strips of sea vegetables (that is, nori, dulse, kombu) to the cooking pot. This enhances digestion, flavor, and nutrient content.

- Other ingredients that can be added: fennel, garlic, onions, cumin seeds, or a little ginger.

- If you must add salt, wait until the beans have softened. This prevents their skins from remaining tough.

- Always ensure that beans are tender and well cooked before eating.

MY FAB FIVE BEANS

A study published in the *Journal of Lipid Research* (June 1997) showed that eating beans regularly lowers cholesterol and prevents heart disease.

1. Adzuki Beans

Adzuki beans are small and red with a sweet peppery flavor. In Japan, they are known as the "king of beans" because of their healing qualities.

Boiled adzuki bean water may be effective for the treatment of kidney and bladder infections, and relieving constipation.[166] Adzuki contains high levels of B vitamins, as well as iron, zinc, and manganese. These beans are the lowest in calories of all beans but contain the highest level of nutrients. I have used these beans with patients who suffer from yeast infections, successfully drying mucus and fungal conditions. Adzuki beans strengthen the spleen as a result of this damp-clearing effect.

2. Mung Beans

Similar in appearance to adzuki with the exception of color (mung beans are green), mung is a popular sprouting bean. Therapeutically, they work to ease water retention and have been shown to lower high blood pressure.[167] Mung beans "tone" the blood; they contain compounds that aid the organs' detoxifying processes.

3. Fava Beans

These are high in B vitamins, calcium, protein, and iron. They are tasty by themselves or added to soups or salads. They have a sweet flavor and are strengthening to the pancreas and spleen. Fava beans have a soft potato-like texture.

4. Soybeans

Due to its complete protein content, the soybean has become a popular alternative to meat. It's also a rich source of essential fatty acids and lecithin, nutrients necessary for brain function and fat emulsification. A beneficial compound known as phytosterols, contained in soy, helps to inhibit the uptake of cholesterol by blocking its absorption.

In research, the consumption of soybeans is now being associated with reduced rates of breast cancer. Findings may be related to the presence of isoflavone compounds that are mildly estrogenic and anticarcinogenic. Soybean products contain several anticancer compounds including phytoestrogen.[168] The effects of soy consumption on circulating hormones was measured in premenopausal women. Results concluded that consumption of soy diets containing phytoestrogens may reduce circulating ovarian steroids and adrenal androgens (male hormones), thus decreasing the risk of breast cancer.[169]

Soybeans can be eaten in their whole form or as tofu or tempeh—two delicious soy-based dishes. Unfortunately, there are many brands of genetically modified soy on the market. Therefore, the best place to buy soy products that are not genetically modified is your health store or natural foods shop. Look for soy products that are certified organic. Soybeans should be consumed in very small amounts. Foods containing soy protein isolates should be avoided as they are highly processed.

5. Lentils

There are over fifty varieties of lentils in different shapes, colors, and sizes. These members of the legume family rate second in protein after soy. The most common lentils are the green, red, and brown varieties—all of which are easy to cook and have a distinct earthy flavor. Your kidneys, adrenal system, and heart should benefit from including lentils in your life.

More Seeds and Nuts

In a nutshell, nuts and seeds contain a powerhouse of nutrients: especially protein, vitamins B and E, and the minerals calcium, magnesium, phosphorus, zinc, iron, potassium, copper, selenium, and manganese. They're also a fine source of essential fatty acids. Because they are such a concentrated food source, nuts and seeds are best eaten in moderation. Add them to desserts, sprinkle them on cereals and salads, or simply eat them as a snack in between meals.

Pumpkin

Characteristically, pumpkin seeds can be recognized by their deep shade of green. They are particularly favored for their high zinc, calcium, B vitamins, and essential fatty acid levels. Eaten regularly, pumpkin seeds can rid the intestinal tract of unwanted parasites.[170]

Sesame

Sesame seeds contain up to 25 percent protein, plus vitamins A, B, and E, and a generous helping of the good fats. As for minerals, they are exceptionally rich in calcium, potassium, iron, magnesium, copper, and zinc. Just 25 g per ounce equals over 1,000 mg of calcium!

Almonds

Almonds have been called the "king of nuts" because of their exceedingly high nutrient content, including potassium, phosphorus, and protein. Many

American cancer clinics are now prescribing ten or more almonds per day, since they are so rich in laetrile. The laetrile has been shown in laboratory animal studies to act as a strong anticancer agent.

Chestnuts

Delicious raw, boiled, or baked, chestnuts are the lowest in fat of all nuts.[171]

Pecans

Pecans are high in potassium, vitamin A, and essential fatty acids. They are excellent for baking and making candy.

Walnuts

Rich in potassium, magnesium, and vitamin A, walnuts are a delicious additions to cakes, biscuits, salads, and dessert toppings.

Other Green Algae

Spirulina

Spirulina is a cultivated or farmed micro-algae, with one of the richest protein contents of all natural foods. By dry weight, it contains 60 percent protein (three times that of meat), of which all essential amino acids are present in a balanced ratio. Unlike other high-protein foods, spirulina is easy to absorb and assimilate. Other constituents included in spirulina: beta-carotene, vitamin B_{12}, gamma-linolenic acid, enzymes, trace minerals, and chlorophyll.

I use spirulina with many patients at my clinic in cases of deficiencies, malabsorption, decreased energy levels, and lowered resistance to infections. Spirulina has been shown to be helpful to the kidneys and enriching to the blood.[172]

Spirulina contains a rich supply of a plant pigment called phyco-cyanin, a protein that has been shown to inhibit the formation of cancer colonies.[173]

Chlorella

Chlorella is a group of single-celled fresh water algae and is one of the oldest forms of life. It is rich in a number of nutrients, including protein, vitamin B_{12}, zinc, iron, chlorophyll, and essential fatty acids (omega-3 variety). It is beneficial for the bowel and intestinal tract. Chlorella has also been shown to be effective in reducing cholesterol in the body and pre-venting atherosclerosis.[174]

Bee Products

Royal jelly, bee pollen, and propolis have exceptional healing powers. They are among the more complete nutrient-dense foods.

Royal Jelly

Murray Blum, M.D., of Louisiana State University, and scientists from the U.S. Department of Agriculture discovered that royal jelly contains an anti-biotic almost a quarter as active as penicillin, but without the side effects. These same researchers also found that royal jelly halts the growth of bac-teria that cause skin infections, like boils, as well as intestinal infections.

Royal jelly is so effective for certain health problems because it is packed with vitamins A, C, D, and E, enzymes, hormones, and eighteen amino acids, and also has antibiotic properties. In my clinical practice, I will often use royal jelly for female patients who have just given birth. The demands of pregnancy, the birth process itself, and breast-feeding deplete the body of nutrients, blood, and energy. Royal jelly comes to the rescue, exerting a strong effect on the glandular system (the hormone- and blood-producing glands, that is, the adrenal glands and spleen). Royal jelly is loaded with B complex vitamins, B_6 (pyridoxine), and a high concentra-tion of B_5 (pantothenic acid). These high levels of B vitamins support limp adrenal function, regulating hormone output, thus lessening fatigue. Some patients call it their "rejuvenator." No wonder the queen bee, nurtured on royal jelly, is 40 to 60 percent larger than the worker bees and lives forty times longer (five to eight years compared with two to six months). Royal jelly is also considered to be a fertility tonic for the reproductive organs due to its content of important hormones.

Bee Pollen

Bee pollen is the "Rolls-Royce" of the bee byproducts. It is a powerhouse of nutrients: 185 in total, including 22 amino acids, 27 minerals, and the full range of vitamins, enzymes, carbohydrates, fats, and hormones. This gold, powder-like material is produced by flowering plants and gathered by bees. Bee pollen, a complete food, nourishes the endocrine and nerv-ous systems, organs, and tissues.

In my practice, I have used bee pollen with some success as an antidote to environmental allergies. I recommend that hay fever sufferers prepare at least one month in advance for the allergy season. My patients start with a tiny crumb of local bee pollen granules and work up to one teaspoon daily. Once the allergy season starts, patients may be advised gradually to increase the granules to two teaspoons daily. This program worked for a woman in her mid-fifties, a long-time sufferer of hay fever and sinusitis. Sinusitis is an inflammation and mucus congestion of the nasal sinuses along with upper respiratory infection. This client has been revisiting me for yearly consultations in preparation for the allergy season. We structured her program with a slow buildup of bee pollen granules, accompanied by minor supporting nutrients. The client no longer suffers the classic headache and earache symptoms. Bee pollen has helped this patient to breathe a sigh of relief.

I have also used bee pollen successfully to help patients fight environmental allergies, chronic infections, prostate enlargement, toxicosis, arteriosclerosis, and nutrient deficiency conditions. It is one of the finest natural remedies.

Propolis

This is a resinous material collected by bees from the buds and bark of mainly poplar and fir trees. The bees use it to coat the entire surface of the hive for sterilization. Any predator entering their domain is stung to death, then embalmed with propolis to prevent decay. Propolis is antibacterial, antiviral, and antiparasitic. Its high concentration of flavonoids may play a protector role in inhibiting bacteria and fungi. Flavonoids also exert a positive effect on the thymus gland, endocrine and adrenal glands, pancreas, cardiovascular system and blood.

Propolis prevents bacteria from multiplying in an organism, and thus has the capability to stimulate the human immune system. Russian surgeons often feed propolis to their patients before surgery as a precaution against infection. Propolis activates the thymus gland, which helps the body to produce its own natural antibiotics.[175] According to Dr. Rémy Chauvin of the Sorbonne, Paris (considered to be the world's leading authority on propolis), the antiviral and antibacterial compounds within propolis improve the body's resistance to infections and thus help to strengthen immunity. Conventional pharmaceutical antibiotics do the opposite. Drug medications, especially when overused, can kill the friendly bacteria in the system: the bacteria needed to maintain a healthy balance. The propolis maintains and enhances the essential healthy bacteria. Its capacity to destroy or halt the multiplication of negative bacteria is helpful in clinical practice. As a result, propolis has been used successfully to improve acne, skin ailments, cold sores, and even arthritis because of its antifungal, antiseptic, and anti-inflammatory qualities.

16.

HOW TO MAKE
MY PROGRAM WORK

QUICK TIPS FOR INSTANT RESULTS

If you implement the five quick tips in this chapter, then you will progress at a much faster rate. When my own patients incorporate these quick tips into my program, they start to experience the benefits almost immediately.

1. Eat slowly—one of the main causes of digestive disorders is unchewed food. Chew it well.

2. Eat simply—we normally eat far too many different competing foods at the same meal, making digestion difficult. It's generally best to eat from no more than one or two different food groups at one meal. For example, protein foods need acid enzyme digestive juices, while carbohydrate foods need alkaline enzyme juices. The effectiveness of both enzyme groups therefore is drastically diminished when foods from both groups need to be broken down at the same time: complete digestion is difficult to obtain. Bloating, gas, heartburn, indigestion, cramps, constipation, and malabsorption often result.

Fruits should be eaten alone as they digest much faster than non-fruit foods. If you try to combine them with dense proteins such as meat, or dense carbohydrates (potatoes or pasta), you will create fermentation in your gut, causing a proliferation of undesirable bacteria.

3. Don't eat food too hot—it can disrupt the digestive enzymes and injure the lining of the stomach; or too cold—it can slow down enzyme action.

4. Drink a cup of warm water in the morning before eating—it goes right to the bowels and cleans mucus out from the day before.

5. Make your meals attractive—this isn't just to give you a psychological boost or to appeal to your artistic nature; it's biochemistry as well. When you see food or smell food or think about food, the brain sends a message to the salivary glands to secrete saliva, which contains the enzyme ptyalin. So attractive meals could actually aid digestion!

THE MCKEITH FOOD GROUPS

The Yes Foods

1. **Vegetables, roots, and live sprouts**

2. **Fruits**

3. **Grains**—such as rice, millet, quinoa, spelt, oats, amaranth, and teff

4. **Beans**—such as kidney, soy, black, lima, marrow, fava, and lentils

5. **Seeds**—such as sunflower, sesame, and pumpkin

6. **Nuts**—such as chestnuts, Brazil, walnuts, hazelnuts, and almonds

7. **Sea vegetables**—such as dulse, nori, wakame, and kombu. Loaded with minerals, vitamins, and enzymes, sea vegetables are excellent when added to soups, casseroles, and savory dishes.

8. **Water**—drink 6–8 glasses a day

9. **Fish**—especially salmon and deep-water fish

10. **Free-range eggs**—in moderation

11. **Yogurts**—(goat, sheep, soy)

12. **Freshly squeezed juices**

See my list of 100+ Right Foods on page 160 for more ideas.

The No Foods: What to Avoid and Why

There are certain bad foods that not only do you no good, but could do you harm. Needless to say, these nasty foods should be avoided, cut out, or at least cut down. These bad foods are coffee, alcohol, caffeine, chocolate, sugar, fatty foods, and refined and processed foods (such as white refined bread, flour, etc.).

Coffee

Coffee contains caffeine, also present in tea and cola drinks. Caffeine is a stimulating drug that negatively acts on the central nervous system (the brain and spinal cord). It can adversely affect the heart, muscles, and digestive juices. It will undo or counteract all the good we are trying to achieve here. Just one cup can cause your blood pressure to rise. When you drink too much coffee, you may become restless, sleepless, anxious, and even experience palpitations because of caffeine's effect on the neurological system. But when you haven't had a cup for a while, you could also exhibit withdrawal symptoms: fatigue, irritability, confusion, headaches, anxiety, even nausea; this is only a further testament to its properties as a drug.

The paradox: although coffee is a stimulant, the end result is fatigue. The adrenal glands produce more stress hormones when you drink caffeine; and these glands then get tired and sluggish from overprocessing caffeine. This can result in weight gain, slowing down of mental processes, memory lapse, and general cell and organ deterioration.

Coffee is also thought to have a serious aging effect on the skin. All coffee, even decaffeinated, contains the chemical benzoic acid. This chemical is essentially toxic; and the body has to neutralize it with an amino acid called glycine before excretion. But glycine also builds and repairs collagen, which keeps the skin firm and wrinkle-free. So if your glycine stores are depleted from neutralizing the benzoic acid in your coffee, what'll be left to stop your skin from sagging into wrinkles? Another problem with coffee (and traditional black tea): it reduces the absorption of iron and zinc by up to 50 percent. Instead, drink a rotation of fruit and herbal teas: peppermint, chamomile, nettle, red clover, red sage, dandelion, for example, or simply fruit juice with hot water.

Fatty Foods

Too many fatty foods can harden the arteries, form excess mucus, and congest and hamper the function of other vital organs. This can lead to high blood pressure, food allergies, heart disease, diabetes, eating disorders, colon congestion, and perhaps cancers. Fatty foods may include certain meats, dairy products, fried foods, and common "junk foods."

Sweets

An excess of sweet foods can cause blood sugar imbalances and hyperactivity. These sugary foods can overwork the spleen, pancreas, liver, and intestines; cause mood swings, irritability, and fatigue; lower resistance to infection; and ultimately lead to hypoglycemia and even diabetes. Avoid refined sugars, corn (maize) syrup, and artificial sweeteners. Honey, molasses, and pure fruit juice—natural sweeteners—can be used at times in moderation, but only very sparingly.

Red Meat

Too many high-protein, fatty red animal foods can toxify and acidify the blood, deplete calcium, overwork the kidneys and liver, and stagnate digestion, destroying the beneficial flora. Several studies confirm that this can ultimately lead to kidney stones, liver fatigue, colon and bowel disorders, constipation, arthritis, osteoporosis, and heart disease.

Cows' Milk and Dairy Foods

Milk is designed for babies and children, not adults. And cows' milk is for calves, not humans. Cows' milk is high in the protein casein. The molecules of casein are too large for humans to digest. Cows' milk also contains at least twenty-five additional proteins in a form and ratio unsuited to humans; these can trigger allergic responses such as sinusitis, asthma, earache, congestion and runny nose, skin rash, eczema, fatigue, lethargy, and irritability. When I remove cows' milk from the diet of allergic patients, most of the common allergic symptoms disappear. Immune response also improves.

Whole cows' milk is too high in saturated fat and low in vitamins and the mineral content is out of balance with human biochemistry; as a result, many of its nutrients cannot be absorbed by humans. Also, cows are normally subjected to hundreds of different drug injections, hormones, pesticides, and drug residues, which in turn make their way into the milk.

Many adults lack the enzyme lactase, which breaks down the lactose sugars in milk. This indigestibility may cause bloating, flatulence, diarrhea, or constipation. In those people with weak digestive function, milk and dairy foods can also cause premenstrual tension, bloating, headaches, irritability, confusion, cramps, allergies, lethargy, sluggish organs, and certain cancers (especially breast cancer).

Alcohol

Alcohol puts a strain on the digestive system and particularly the liver. The liver converts alcohol into acetaldehyde, a toxic cousin of formaldehyde used in tanning leather and the embalming process. Overuse of alcohol can lead to *Candida albicans,* hypoglycemia, diabetes, fatigue, sluggish organs, and cell tissue degeneration.

FOOD COMBINING

Food combining is not a theory. Rather it is biochemistry and physiology. Food combining dramatically helps your digestion. It ensures that you absorb the maximum nutrients from food. In effect, when you combine foods properly, you prevent contradictory digestive enzymes from competing with each other.

The Problem

If you eat too many different food groups at the same time you

1. make complete digestion impossible,

2. upset digestive enzymes,

3. prevent nutrient uptake, and

4. risk a host of ills including bloating, heartburn, indigestion, malabsorption, constipation, cramps, flatulence or worse.

   The problem is that some foods are digested more quickly than others, some need different digestive enzymes, and others need different conditions in the stomach for good digestion. Proteins need acid digestive juices, while carbohydrates need alkaline juices for their digestion. When my own patients at the clinic embark upon my food combining methods, they often notice significant improvements within just a few days. My program not only eradicates bloating, heartburn, indigestion, constipation, irritable bowel syndrome, migraines, malabsorption, and gas with food combining, but my patients report greater energy levels and elevated moods and overall vitality. Biochemical enzyme testing at the clinic also proves enhanced or corrected digestive activity after food combining.

The Situation

Group 1—Proteins (meat, poultry, cheese, fish, eggs, milk, nuts) produce acid juices for their digestion. They digest slowly.

Group 2—Carbohydrates (all grains and the foods made from them—bread, pasta, cereals, flour, biscuits etc. and starchy vegetables—potatoes, yams, sweet corn) produce alkaline juices. They digest quickly and require different enzymes. If you eat these groups together, you will cause a digestive battle of competing enzymes. The result is that the food doesn't get digested properly. Hence the gas, bloating, heartburning stomach pains, malabsorption, indigestion, and energy drain.

Group 3—Salads, non-starchy vegetables, roots, seeds, herbs, spices, nut and seed oils can be digested with either Group 1 or Group 2.

Group 4—Fruit is out on its own. It holds the record for the fastest digestion rate. Fruit uses completely different enzymes from all other groups.

The Solution

- Don't eat Group 1 (proteins) and Group 2 (carbohydrates) together at the same meal.

- Group 3 (vegetables) can be eaten with Groups 1 or 2.

- Group 4 (fruit) must always be eaten on its own, at least thirty minutes away from other food groups. It's best to eat fruit on an empty stomach, preferably in the morning with no other food types. If you eat fruit after a meal, it will ferment in the gut. It can't go anywhere, because it's stuck behind food that takes much longer to digest. When fruit is indeed mixed with other food groups, you might expect bloating, flatulence, indigestion. (Never mix melons with other fruits. Melons digest the fastest of all fruits. Therefore, eat alone or leave alone!)

- Leave two hours after a carbohydrate meal before eating protein. Leave three hours after a protein meal before eating carbohydrates. Protein takes four hours to reach the bowel, and carbohydrate meals take two hours from mouth to bowel.

See the following chart for more details of the different food groups.

DIFFERENT FOOD GROUPS		
Group 1 **Proteins**	**Group 2** **Carbohydrates**	**Group 3** **Greens and non-** **starchy vegetables**
Dried beans	Grains, including oats, pasta, rice, rye, maize, millet	Salads and fresh herbs
Dried peas		Seeds
Cheese	Grain products, biscuits, bread, cakes, crackers, and pastry	Sprouts
Nuts		Vegetable spreads
Eggs (free-range)	Honey	Olive oil (cold pressed)
Fish	Maple syrup	Herbs, spices, and seasonings
Game/rabbit	Potatoes and starchy vegetables (e.g., yams, chestnuts, squash, lima beans, pumpkins, parsnips)	
Meat		Nut and seed oils
Milk		Algae
Poultry		
Shellfish		
Soybeans, tofu and all soy products, miso soup		
Yogurt		

Follow my chart and improve your digestion, energy, stamina, and join the path to perfect health.

Food Combining Chart

BAD BOX
Grain with dairy or meat = Gas
Fruit and vegetables = Gas
Fruit and meats = Gas
Fruit with grain or dairy = Gas

GOOD BOX
Fruit by itself = NO Gas, proper digestion
Grain with vegetables = NO Gas
Pasta with vegetables = NO Gas
Beans with vegetables = NO Gas
Fish with vegetables = NO Gas

DR. GILLIAN'S TOP 100+ RIGHT FOODS

Just when you thought there was nothing left to eat, here's my list of the best foods to include in your life.

LEAFY GREEN VEGETABLES

Arugula

Beet greens

Chicory

Collards

Dandelion greens

Endive

Escarole

Iceberg lettuce

Kale

Loose-leaf lettuce

Mâche

Mustard greens

Parsley

Romaine

Sorrell

Spinach

Swiss chard

Turnip greens

Watercress

VEGETABLES

Artichoke

Asparagus

Avocado

Beetroot

Broccoli

Brussels sprouts

Cabbage: bok choy

Chinese cabbage

Carrots

Cauliflower

Celeriac

Celery

Daikon

Eggplant

Green peas

Kohlrabi

Okra

Onions

Parsnips

Peppers

Potatoes

Radish

Squash

Tomatoes

Turnip

Yams

Zucchini

SEA VEGETABLES (SEAWEEDS)

Agar

Arame

Dulse

Hijiki

Kelp

Kombu

Nori

Sea palm

Wakame

RAW NUTS

Almonds

Brazil nuts

Hazelnuts

Chestnuts

Pecans

Pine nuts

Pistachios

Walnuts

FRUIT

Acid Fruits

Cranberries

Currants

Dates

Gooseberries

Grapefruit

Kumquat

Lemons

Limes

Loganberries

Oranges

Passion fruit

Pineapples

Pomegranates

Strawberries

Tangelos

Tangerines

Sub-Acid

Apples

Apricots

Blackberries

Blueberries

Cherries

Grapes

Guava

Huckleberries

Kiwi

Litchi

Loquat

Mango

Mulberries

Nectarine

Papaya

Peach

Pear

Prickly pears (cactus fruit)

Sweet Fruits

Banana

Dates

Figs

Dried fruit

Persimmon

Plantain

Melons

Banana melon

Honeydew melon

Watermelon

FRESH HERBS

(For seasoning)

Basil

Bay leaves

Cardamom

Chervil

Cinnamom

Cloves

Coriander

Cumin

Dill

Fennel

Fenugreek

Ginger

Marjoram

Mint

Oregano

Rosemary

Saffron

Tarragon

Thyme

Umeboshi plums

GRAINS

Amaranth

Barley

Buckwheat

Bulgur wheat

Corn

Kamut

Millet

Oats

Quinoa

Basmati rice

Brown rice

Rye

Spelt

FLOURS

Amaranth

Durum wheat

Graham

Jerusalem artichoke

Oat

Potato

Soy

Sunflower seed

Tapioca

BEANS

Adzuki

Anasazi

Black turtle

Fava

Garbanzo

Great Northern

Lentils

Lima

Navy

Pinto

Soy

SEEDS

Chia

Flax

Pumpkin

Sesame

Sunflower

TOFU

TEMPEH

FISH

HERBAL TEAS

Chamomile

Dandelion

Fennel

Ginger

Ginseng

Hawthorn

Horsetail

Lemon balm

Licorice

Melissa

Nettle

Pau d'Arco

Peppermint

Red clover

Red raspberry

Rose-hips

Slippery elm

Spearmint

Valerian root

17.

FINAL SONG
AND DANCE

MOTHERS AND DAUGHTERS

For years and years, since healthy living has been a way of life for me, I have been trying to convert my parents into the fold. It's the natural tendency of a loving daughter, I'm told. I think this is a universal problem. My mother-in-law says she has been trying to convert my father-in-law for the past twenty-two years. "It's not easy," she sighs. I have patients who have been trying to influence their teenage children. I have young patients trying to persuade their parents to adopt a healthy lifestyle; sisters who want to change brothers; brothers trying to change wives. And so on. In the end, we each need to take responsibility for our own lives.

Nonetheless, I keep trying, as God only knows. But to say that my mum is the most traditional conservative Scottish lady in the western hemisphere would be a gross understatement. Set in her ways, there is a very limited repertoire of foods that my mum will eat. They usually have to be words like, or least sound like, shepherd's pie, meat, potatoes, porridge, oatmeal, tea, sugar, custard, and that just about covers it. Well, maybe I'm being a bit unfair! But I remember the time when I was preparing a lovely tofu casserole, and she walked by the cooker moaning "What's that rubbish in the pot?" The truth is that we all have to contend with a loved one who is not ready or willing to make food or lifestyle changes. There's only one solution: live and let live. It is not my obligation, nor yours, to try to convert another person. Surely we each have a responsibility to share our knowledge, but that is where the effort ends. We need not push, pressurize, or pounce on others to adopt our way. Just put it out there into the world, and miracles do occur.

Last year, I received a call from mum in the hospital. She had been heavily medicated, treated, and administered with every imaginable gory test to ascertain a diagnosis of diverticulitis (ironically, a condition caused by poor diet!). For the first time in my life, mum sounded scared, feeble, frighteningly vulnerable, and in pain. She had been hospitalized for attacks of this diverticulitis several previous times, but did not want me to know. This time was different, however. Shaking with fever, torturous stomach pain, and nausea—I'm sure mum thought the end was near. I could feel the fear pulsating through the telephone line. "Gillian, I need your help, please," she softly cried. And I cried too. Mum was finally willing to listen.

Imagine the frustration I had felt when I was helping scores of people at my clinic, but was denied the opportunity to help my own mum suffering from a poor food-induced illness. This particular attack, however, would once and for all quash the song and dance between mother and daughter. I think at last we both just saw each other as adults. The mutual love and kindness has always been there, but now there was a new respect for each other.

A few days later and out of hospital, mum called me again confirming a request for help. I have learned not to push. The patient (or your own mum for that matter) has to want the treatment more than you do. I could not wait to design her a food program specifically for diverticulitis: no dairy (milk), no meats, no fried foods, no sugar—all the things she loved, but now needed to eliminate, or at least reduce.

I put her on aloe vera juice twice daily, flax seed oil, wild blue-green algae, enzymes, and my living food powder. I am pleased to report that my mother has had no attacks of diverticulitis since embarking upon this living food program—for six months thus far. I am convinced that if she stays on the program, she should never experience such ill fate again.

The fact is that living foods can help your parents, your child, your spouse, your friend, your brother, or your sister. But most important, living foods can first help you.

SONG

So I do hope that you will sing the praises of living foods every single day. And in the spirit of song, one of my final words of wisdom is to advise you to sing before and after meals. When you sing, the diaphragm opens, and allows more oxygen to the area. The diaphragm is located alongside the digestive organs. The infusion of oxygen into the diaphragm region relaxes and nourishes the entire area, including the digestive organs. Thus, the digestive organs also become more relaxed, less tense, and far more receptive to the digestion process. As a result, you absorb more nutrients from the foods that you eat and are better able to break down cellulose, starch, and fats. A healthier, calmer, and happier you can emerge.

AND DANCE

In addition to song, I recommend that you dance (or run on the spot) to your favorite music for just a few minutes or more every few hours each day. You can dance during coffee breaks at work, just before lunch, and so on. If you're at home, there's no excuse to not dance. Turn on the radio or CD and go crazy—boogie away. Dancing is one of the most efficient forms of exercise, as it gently works almost every muscle and organ of the body! Dancing also helps to distribute nutrients, improves blood circulation, relieves toxins via sweat, strengthens the heart, gets rid of the "cobwebs" from the brain, and makes you feel tingly all over. Fitness regimens need not be painful, boring, or tedious. Instead, exercise should be easy, gentle and lots of fun—just like dancing. Better yet, how about singing while you dance. See how much fun you can have—so get to it, and most important, enjoy it!

BRING IN THE LIGHT

Finally, my best advice is to thoroughly enjoy the singing and the dancing, and happy eating too, but to also enjoy everything else in life as well. In other words, "allow the Light" to come into your life. This means that I want you to consciously direct feelings of joy, calm, peace, goodness, happiness and all positivity to flow through every cell and every organ in your body. When we consciously and deliberately give clear direct messages to our bodies, the body listens and responds accordingly. Every cell and organism is a dynamic and intelligently responsive creature with vibrational energies. Therefore, our conscious directions can greatly influence the biochemical, physiological, psychological, emotional, metaphysical, and spiritual outcomes.

For example, the Alexander Technique is a century-old English treatment for backaches, poor posture, and improper spinal use. Followers of the technique have found that by literally talking to the spine, disks, and vertebrae, there are significant physical changes that might occur in the back-neck-spinal alignment. People with histories of backaches have experienced relief from pain and shifts in the spinal cord, simply by giving verbal instructions to the back. I can attest to this firsthand. The back listens and then responds with often dramatic improvements.

Similarly, and perhaps not so esoterically, consider the example of when you're on the motorway and a massive traffic jam appears just ahead. Some people may look at the pile-up and immediately react with upset, anger, disappointment, even rage. You might say: "This lousy traffic—I'm sick of these roads. I hate driving." And so on. Your body listens and responds. Soon enough, your palms may get sweaty; you may feel tremors or palpitations; headaches, or even migraines, develop. There you are just about to join a horrendous traffic jam, feeling horrible. This upset causes your blood sugar to fluctuate violently, nutrients to become depleted, and bowels and arteries to tighten, taxing the adrenal glands, and the organs suffer too. You indeed suggested that all this was making you "sick," and it has. Your body listens to what you tell it.

In the meantime, you suddenly notice that what you thought was a massive traffic jam is nothing of the sort; a small insignificant obstacle perhaps, caused a very brief slowdown. The traffic starts flowing again, and you never really had to join any jam after all. But that's irrelevant now, because you truly feel physically terrible from the emotional distress you caused to yourself. In essence, you reacted to the situation! You gave your body and mind nothing but negative input, and your body listened and then responded handsomely to the negativity.

So even though the traffic started to flow freely, your body became more shocked, jammed tight. You failed to "allow the Light" to come in.

If our bodies respond so fluidly to the negative input, imagine how well the body will respond to positive input. We've all heard those stories about how prayer cured this one or that one from some disease. I don't doubt these stories. Prayer is one of the most positive introspective ways to "allow in the Light." Similarly, some of you may have seen the film *Patch Adams,* starring Robin Williams, about the medical doctor who treated patients with laughter therapy. I actually interviewed the real Patch Adams many years ago on the radio. I found his therapy, of encouraging people to laugh, to be another lighting rod for positivity. Any measure that promotes happiness, joy, kindness, goodness, and any other positiveness, is good for us and good for our universe. I tell my husband that the most important thing to me is simply that he is happy. It doesn't take much to please me. Just be happy!

The concept of injecting positive input into all daily life is what I mean by "allowing in the Light." It has far-reaching implications. First, when you shop for food, as an example, allow the Light to come in. Walk through the produce aisle and seek out those fruits and vegetables that convey the strongest energetic and vibrational fields. In other words, what do you desire? What fruits and vegetables seem to be the happiest or the healthiest? This is how you can make choices. We do it every day already at the market on a more physical superficial level. Watch the consumers squeeze the peaches for softness or closely examine the apples for blemished skins. Those fruits that don't make the mark are thrown back into the box. I just want you to take this one step further. Even close your eyes for a one-minute moment of relaxation or meditation before entering the supermarket, and see if you can then better absorb such vibrational fields from the food itself. Which foods "speak" to you?

Next, when you get the food home and prepare it, do so with love and kindness. A plethora of studies and research papers have been written to support the claim that the "energies from the chef can be picked up by the eater." If the food preparer is in a foul mood, this can emotionally contaminate the person eating the food. Conversely, children are emotionally, psychologically, and spiritually nourished (and physically too) when mum or dad is in the kitchen tenderly, happily, and willingly preparing a meal; the loving energy flows to the kids. This is one reason why mum's "home cooking" has such warm appeal! Marketing companies have known this secret for years as they use phraseology like "homestyle," "home-made," "home-grown," "like grandma's cooking," and so forth.

Once the meal is brought to the table, again "allow the Light" to come in. For my own family, this usually means rendering appreciation and thanks for the food. Sometimes we'll have full discussions at the dinner table, recollecting and retracing the possible movements of the food and its ultimate destination with us. We'll thank the seeds, the sun, the rain, the farmers, the transporters, the warehousers, and the shopkeepers for their roles! But somehow we seem to always start and end with God. To me, this represents the truest sense of "letting in the Light": love and a higher force are what it's all about. And by the way, all this positivity at the dinner table is absorbed by the food itself, then into you. The implications of "allowing in the Light" continue on and on indefinitely. In the end, it is all about not reacting with negativity, but rather being proactive and positive and keeping out the darkness. So now I feel complete to sign off for the time being, wishing you all Love and Light!

For nutritional and biochemical testing, contact
www.drgillianmckeith.com

NOTES

1. Cichoke, A., *Enzymes and Enzyme Therapy*, Keats Publishing, Connecticut, 1994, p. 5.

2. Ibid, p. 6.

3. Gascoigne, S., *The Manual of Conventional Medicine for Alternative Practitioners*, Jigme Press, Dorking, Surrey, 1993, p. 255.

4. Ibid

5. McKeith, G., *The Miracle Superfood: Wild Blue-Green Algae*, Keats Publishers, Los Angeles, 1997, p. 44.

6. Szekely, E. B., *The Chemistry of Youth*, US International Biogenic Society, 1977, paper 1–10.

7. Szekely, E. B., "The essene way," *Journal of Biogenic Living*, US International Biogenic Society, 1978.

8. Kenton, L., *The New Biogenic Diet*, Vermilion Press, London 1995, p. 84.

9. Maiser, A. M. and Poljakoff-Mayber, A., *The Germination of Seeds*, Pergammon Press, Oxford, 1989 (4th ed), p. 27.

10. Meyerwitz, S., *Sprouts: The Miracle Food*, Sproutman Publications, Massachusetts, 1998, p. 93.

11. Kenton, *The New Biogenic Diet*, p. 85.

12. Wigmore, A., *The Hippocrates Diet and Health Program*, Avery Publishing, New York, 1984, p. 92.

13. Kenton, *The New Biogenic Diet*, p. 85

14. Wigmore, *The Hippocrates Diet*, p. 97.

15. Ibid, pp. 90–7

16. Ibid, pp. 90–7

17. Meyerowitz, *Sprouts: The Miracle Food*, p. 97.

18. Maiser and Polijakoff-Mayber, *The Germination of Seeds*, p. 27.

19. Haas, E., *Staying Healthy With Nutrition*, Celestial Arts, Berkeley, CA, 1992, p. 319.

20. Wigmore, *The Hippocrates Diet*, p. 72.

21. Tsai, C. Y. and Dalby, A., "Lysine and tryptophane increases during germination of maize seeds," *Journal of Cereal Chemistry*, Purdue University, vol. 52, no. 3, 1975.

22. Wigmore, *The Hippocrates Diet*, p. 72.

23. Ibid, pp. 73–4.

24. Cousens, G., *Spiritual Nutrition and the Rainbow Diet*, Cassandra Press, San Rafael, California, 1986, p. 104.

25. Kenton, *The New Biogenic Diet*, p. 86.

26. Fahey, J. W., Yueshing, Z. and Talalay, P., Anti-cancer properties of sprout extracts," Proceedings of the National Academy of Sciences, Johns Hopkins Medical School, Baltimore, MD, 16 September 1997.

27. "Researchers find a concentrated anti-cancer substance," *New York Times*, 16 September 1997.

28. Kushi, M., *The Macrobiotic Way*, Avery Publishing, New York, 1993, p. 65.

29. Pitchford, P., *Healing with Whole Foods*, North Atlantic Books, Berkely, CA, 1993, p. 529.

30. Holmes, P., *The Energetics of Herbs*, Snow Lotus Press, Colorado, 1997, pp. 436–8.

31. Foster, S., *Herbs For Your Health*, Interweave Press, Colorado, 1996, p. 2.

32. Ritchason, J., *The Little Herb Encyclopaedia*, Woodland Health Books, Utah, 1996, p. 2.

33. Holmes, *The Energetics of Herbs*, p. 436.

34. McKeith, G., *10 Steps to Perfect Health for All Mothers*, Lowell House, Los Angeles, 2000 (forthcoming).

35. Holmes, *The Energetics of Herbs*, pp. 436–8.

36. Bradley, B. A., "Uses of alfalfa," *Observation with Medicago Sativa*, Lloyd Brothers, Cincinnati, Ohio, 1915. Reprinted in Foster, *Herbs for Your Health*, p. 2.

37. Lorenzetti, L. J. et al., "Bacteriostactic property of aloe vera," *Journal of Pharmacological Science*, vol. 53, 1964, p. 1287.

38. Hegger, J. P., Pineless, G. R. and Robson, M. C., "Dermaide aloe/aloe vera gel: comparison of the antimicrobial effects," *Journal of American Medical Technology*, no. 41, 1979, pp. 293–4.

39. Stepanova, O. S. et al., "Chemical composition and biological activity of dry aloe leaves," *Fiziol, Aktivnye Vesh*, No. 9, 1997, pp. 94–7.

40. Sims, R. M. and Zimmerman, E. R., "The effect of aloe vera on mycotic organism (fungi)," *Aloe Vera of America Archives, Stabilized Aloe Vera*, vol. 1, 1971, pp. 237–8.

41. Bland, J., "Effect of orally consumed aloe vera juice on human gastrointestinal function," *Natural Foods Network Newsletter*, August 1985. Also printed in *Preventive Medicine*, March/April 1985.

42. Womble and Helderman, "Enhancement of allo-responsiveness of human lymphocytes by acemannan," *International Journal of Immuno Pharmacology*, vol.10, no. 8, 1988, pp. 967–74.

43. Plaskett, L., "The healing properties of aloe vera," *Biomedical Information Services Ltd*, no. 4, 1996, p. 3.

44. Afzal, M. et al., "Identification of some protanoids in aloe vera extracts," *Planta Medica*, no. 57, 1991, p. 364.

45. Pitchford, *Healing With Whole Foods*, p. 364.

46. McIntyre, A., "The virgin healer," *Healthy Eating Magazine*, Market Link, Saffron Walden, Essex, 1995.

47. Sims, R. M. and Zimmerman, E. R., "The effect of aloe vera on herpes simplex and herpes virus (strain: zoster)," *Aloe Vera of America Archives, Stabilized Aloe Vera*, vol. 1, 1971, pp. 239–40.

48. Blitz, J. J., Smith, J. W. and Gerard, R. R., "Aloe vera gel in peptic ulcer therapy: preliminary report," *American Osteopathology Society*, no. 62, 1963, pp. 731–5.

49. Rubel, B. L., *Possible Mechanisms of the Healing Actions of Aloe Gel,* Cosmet Toiletries, 1983, no. 98, pp.109–14.

50. Bunyapraphatsara, N. et al., "Antidiabetic activity of aloe vera L juice II. Clinical trial in diabetes mellitus patients in combination with glibenclamede," *Phytomedicine,* vol. 3, no. 3, 1996, pp. 245–8.

51. El Zawahry, M., Heagazy, M. R. and Helal, M., "Use of aloe in treating leg ulcers and dermatoses," *Int. of Dermatology,* no. 12, 1973, pp. 68–73.

52. Sheets, M. A. et al., "Studies of the effect of acemannan (tradename) on retrosirius infections: clinical stabilization of feline leukaemia virus-infected cats," *Molecular Biother,* no. 3 (1), 1991, pp. 41–5.

53. Plaskett, L., "Aloe against infections," *Biomedical Information Services Ltd,* Issue 9, 1996, p. 6.

54. Kahlon, J. B. et al., "In vitro evaluation of the synergistic antiviral effects of acemannan in combination with azidothymidine and acyclovir," *Molecular Biother,* no. 3, 1991, pp. 214–24.

55. Kahlon, J. B., Kemp, M. C. and Carpenter, R. H., "Inhibition of aids virus replication by acemannan in vitro," *Molecular Biother,* no. 3, 1991, pp. 127–35.

56. Seibold, R. L., *Cereal Grasses,* Keats Publishing, Connecticut, 1996, p. 12.

57. Lee, W. H., Preface in Yoshihide, Hagiwara, MD, *Green Barley Essence,* Keats Publishing, Connecticut, 1996.

58. Hagiwara, Yoshihide, *Green Barley Essence,* Keats Publishing, Connecticut, 1996.

59. Osawa, T. et al., "A novel antioxidant isolated from young green barley leaves," *Journal of Agricultural Food Chemistry,* no. 40, 1978, pp. 1135–8.

Iboh, T. and Tsukagoshi, S., "Study on the anticancer activity of green juice powder of gramincac plants," The 98th Annual Assembly of the Pharmaceutical Society of Japan, 1979. Published in Badamchian, M., "Isolation of a vitamin E analog from a green barley leaf extract," *The Journal of Nutritional Biochemistry,* vol. 5, Washington, DC, March 1994, p. 148.

60. Seibold, *Cereal Grasses,* p. 12

61. Ibid, p. 16.

62. Ibid, p. 15.

63. Hagiwara, *Green Barley Essence,* p.4.

64. Lai, C., Butler, M. and Matney, T. M., "Antimutagenic activities of common vegetables and their chlorophyll content," *Mutation Research,* 77, pp. 245–50.

65. Hagiwara, *Green Barley Essence,* p.2

66. Seibold, *Cereal Grasses,* pp. 20–3.

67. Heinerman, J., Foreword in Seibold, *Cereal Grasses.*

68. Hagiwara, *Green Barley Essence,* pp. 74, 135.

69. Ohtake, et al. (Research Laboratory, Science University of Tokyo), "Studies on the constituents of green juice from young barley leaves, antiulcer activity of fractions from barley juice," *Yakaguka Zasshi,* vol. 105, no. 11, 1985, pp. 1046–51.

70. Pitchford, *Healing with Whole Foods,* Part II: Essentials of Nutrition, p. 200.

71. Kazuhiko, et al., "Isolation of potent anti-inflammatory protein from barley leaves," *Japanese Journal of Inflammation,* vol. 3, no. 4, 1983, pp. 1–3.

72. Ibid

73. Ibid, pp. 1–3.

74. Pitchford, *Healing with Whole Foods,* Part II: Essentials of Nutrition, pp. 199–200.

75. Whitaker, J., *Health and Healing,* vol. 6, no. 7, July 1996, p. 2.

76. Dyerberg, J., Bang, H. O. and Hjorne, N., "Fatty acid composition of plasma lipids in Greenland Eskimos," *American Journal of Clinical Nutrition,* no. 28, 1975, pp. 958–66

77. Johnston, I. M. and Johnston, J. R., *Flaxseed (Linseed) Oil and the Power of Omega-3,* Keats Publishing, Connecticut, 1990.

78. De Lorgeril, M., et al., "Trial: Mediterranean alpha-linolenic acid-rich diet in secondary prevention of coronary heart disease," *The Lancet,* vol. 343, 1994, pp. 1454–9.

79. Renaud, S. and Nordoy, A., "Small is beautiful: a linolenic acid," *The Lancet,* vol. 1, 1983, p. 1169.

80. Thompson, L. U., Robb, P., Serraino, M. and Cheung, F., "Mammalian lignan production from various foods," *Journal of Nutrition and Cancer,* vol. 16, 1991, p. 43.

81. Serraino, M. and Thompson, L. U., "Flaxseed supplementation and early markers of colon carcinogenesis," *Cancer Letters,* vol. 63, 1992, p. 159.

82. Adlercretuz, H., "Does fiber-rich food containing animal lignan precursors protect against both colon and breast cancer? An extension of the 'Fiber hypothesis'," *Gastroenterology,* vol. 86, 1984, p. 761.

83. Kurzer, M., Slavin, J. and Adlercreutz, H., "Flaxseed, lignans and sex hormones," Department of Food Science and Nutrition, University of Minnesota, USA and Department of Clinical Chemistry, University of Helsinki, Finland, 1992, pp. 136–44.

84. Kurzer, M., Lampe, J., Martini, M. and Adlercreutz, H., "Fecal lignan and isoflavonoid excretion in premenopausal women consuming flaxseed powder," *Cancer Epidemiology, Biomarkers and Prevention,* vol. 4, June 1995, pp. 353–8.

85. Phipps, W. R., Lampe, M. C., Slavin, J. L. and Kurzer, M., "Effect of flaxseed ingestion on the menstrual cycle," *Journal of Clinical Endocrinology Metabolism,* vol. 77, 1993, pp. 1215–19.

86. Haggerty, W., "Flax, ancient herb and modern medicine," *Herbalgram Magazine,* vol. 45, American Botanical Council, Austin, Texas, Winter 1999, p. 53.

87. Axelson, M., Sjovall, J., Gustafsson, B. E. and Setchell, K. D. R., "Origin of lignans in mammals and identification of a precursor from plants," *Nature,* no. 298, 1982, pp. 659.

88. Booriello, S. P., Setchell, K. D., Axelson, M. and Lauson, A. M., "Production and metabolism of lignans by the human fecal flora," *J. Apple. Bacterial.,* no. 58, pp. 37.

89. Fisher, W. L., *How to Fight Cancer and Win,* Alive Books, Vancouver, Canada, 1987, p. 57.

90. Ibid, p. 78.

91. Dickinson, A. and Scherer, R. P., "Survey of health and nutrition literature," *Omega-3 Fatty Acids Review,* June 1988, pp. 1–5.

92. Murray, M., and Pizzorno, J., *Encyclopedia of Natural Medicine,* Prima Health, California, 1998, p. 533.

93. Werback, M., *Nutritional Influences on Illness, A Sourcebook of Clinical Research,* Keats Publishing, New Canaan, Connecticut, 1987, pp. 67–416.

94. Cunnane, C. S., "High linolenic acid flaxseed (*Linum usitatissimum*): some nutritional properties in humans," *British Journal of Nutrition,* vol. 69, 1993, pp. 443–53.

95. Swanson, M., "Alpha-linolenic acid," *Townsend Letter For Doctors and Patients,* Townsend Letter Group, Townsend, Washington, October 1998, p. 55.

96. Horrobin, D. F. et al., "Abnormalities in plasma essential fatty acid levels in women with premenstrual syndrome and with non-malignant breast disease," *Journal of Nutritional Medicine,* vol. 2, 1991, pp. 259–64.

Bougnoux, P. et al., "Linolenic acid content of adipose breast tissue: a host determinant of the risk of early metastasis in breast cancer," *British Journal of Cancer,* no. 70, 1994, p. 330.

97. Brenner, R. R., "Nutritional and hormonal factors influencing desaturation of essential fatty acids," *Prog. Lipid Research,* no. 20, 1982, pp. 41–4.

Boyd, N. F., McGuire, V., Shannon, P. et al., "Effect of low-fat, high carbohydrate diet on symptoms of clinical mastopathy," *The Lancet,* vol. 2, 1988, pp. 128–32.

98. Kowalchiki, C. and Hylton, W. (eds), *Rodale's Illustrated Encyclopedia of Herbs,* Rodale Press, Pennsylvania, 1987, p. 407.

99. Prakash, D. et al., "Parsley extracts and anti-fungal activity," *Fitotherapia,* no. 51, 1980, p. 285.

100. Sollman, T., *A Manual of Pharamacology,* 7th ed., W. B. Saunders, Philadelphia, 1948, p. 148.

101. Murphy, E. W., March, A. C. and Willis, B. W., "Nutrient content of spices and herbs," *Journal of the American Dietetic Association,* 1978, pp. 72, 174–6.

102. Duke, J., *CRC Handbook of Medicinal Herbs,* CRC Press Inc., Boca Raton, Florida, 1985, p. 357.

103. Tanaka, Y., "The binding of lead by a Pacific polyelectrolyte," *Environmental Research,* no. 14, 1977, pp. 126–40.

104. Tanaka, Y., "Studies on inhibition of intestinal absorption of radio-active strontium," *Canadian Medical Association Journal,* no. 99, 1968, pp. 169–75.

105. McConnaughey, E., *Sea Vegetables,* Naturegraph Publishers, California, 1985, p. 45.

106. USDA and Japan Nutritonist Association Food Tables, Gerras, C. (ed.), *Rodale's Basic Natural Foods Cookbook,* Rodale Press, Emmaus, Pennsylvania, 1984, p. 249.

107. Abe, S. and Keaneda, T., "The effect of edible seaweeds on cholesterol metabolism in rats," Proceedings of the 7th International Seaweed Symposium, Japan, Department of Food Chemistry, Tohoku University, Japan, August 1971, p. 562.

108. Pitchford, *Healing With Whole Foods,* p. 544.

109. Ibid, p. 552.

110. Elkins, R., *Stevia, Nature's Sweetner,* Woodland Publishing, Utah, pp. 18, 21.

111. Ibid, 22

112. Ibid, 21

113. Kinghorn, A. D. and Soejarto, D. D., "Current status of stevioside as a sweetening agent for human use," *Economic and Medicinal Plant Research,* vol. 1, Academia Press Incorporated, Chicago, IL, 1985, pp. 30, 38.

Melis, M. S., "A crude extract of *Stevia rebaudiana* increases the renal plasma flow of normal and hypertensive rats," *Brazilian Journal of Medical Research,* vol. 29, no. 5, 1996, pp. 669–75.

Melis, M. S., "Chronic administration of aqueous extract of *Stevia rebaudiana* in rats: renal effects," *Journal of Ethnopharmacology,* vol. 47, no. 3, 1995, pp. 129–34.

114. Elkins, *Stevia, Nature's Sweetner,* p. 12.

115. Slagle, P., *The Way Up From Down,* Random Books, New York, 1987, pp. 30–5.

116. Oviedo, C. A., Fronciani, G., Moreno, R. Y. and Maas, L. C., (Hospital Universitario, Paraguay), "Hypoglycaemic action of *Stevia rebaudiana bertoni,*" *Excerpta Media,* no. 209, 1970, p. 92.

117. Curl, et al., "Effect of *Stevia rebaudiana* on glucose tolerance in normal adult humans," *Brazilian Journal of Medical Bioliogical Research,* vol. 19, 1986, pp. 771–4.

118. Vignas, P. V., Duee, E. D., Vignais, P. M. and Nuet, J., *Biochemica et Biophysica Acta,* no. 118, pp. 465–71.

119. Bracht, K., "Hypoglcemic effect of *Stevia rebaudiana:* inhibition of gluconeogenesis in isolated renal tubules," Proceedings of the 18th Congress of the Sociedade Brasileira de Fisiologia, *Brazilian Journal of Medical Biological Research,* vol. 16, nos. 5 and 6, Paraná, Brazil, 1983, 52.2.

120. Rogers, S., *The Cure Is In The Kitchen,* Prestige Publishing, New York, 1990, p. 73.

121. Elkins, *Stevia, Nature's Sweetner,* p. 9, 26.

122. Miguel, O., "A new aural hypoglycemite," *Medical Review of Paraguay* 8, nos. 5 and 6, July–Dec 1966, p. 200.

123. Whitaker, J., *Health and Healing Newsletter,* Phillips Publishing Inc., December 1994, pp. 1–5.

124. Pinheiro, C. et al., "Effect of *Stevia rebaudiana bertoni* (leaves) extracts and stevioside, on the fermentation and synthesis of extracellular insoluble polysaccharides of dental plaque," *Orthodontic Review Journal,* University of Sao Paulo, vol. 1, no. 4, 1987, p. 9–13.

125. Bonvie, L., Bonvie B. and Gates, D., *The Stevia Story,* B.E.D., Atlanta, GA, 1977, pp. 7–10.

126. Ibid, pp. 15–25.

127. Ibid, p. 47.

128. Ibid, pp. 55–60.

129. Ensminger, *Foods and Nutrition Encyclopedia,* vol. 2, no. 1–2, Pegus Press, Clovis, CA, 1983 1st ed., p. 2074.

Food and Nutrition Newsletter, Rodale Press, Summer, 1983, p. 24.

130. *Alive,* Issue 175

131. *Herbal Health Products*—www.viable.com/sunflow.htm

Shannon, S., *Diet for the Atomic Age,* Avery Publishing Group, Inc., Wayne, New Jersey, 1987, p. 156.

132. Prottey, C., Hartop, P., and Press, M., "Correction of the cutaneous manifestations of essential fatty acid deficiency in man by application of sunflower seed oil to the skin," *The Journal of Investigative Dermatology,* no. 64, 1975, pp. 228–34.

133. "The effect of olive oil and sunflower oils on low density lipoprotein level, composition, size, oxidisation and interaction with arterial proteoglycans," *Phytochemistry,* December 1996.

134. Fay, P., "The blue-greens (*Cyanophyta-cyanobacteria*)," *The Institute of Biology's Studies in Biology,* no. 160, Edward Arnold, London, 1983, pp. 1–3

135. France, R., *The Miracle of Blue-Green Algae,* in association with CellTech Publications, Klamath Falls, 1994, p. 39.

136. Michael, J., "Wild blue-green algae: from power to promise," in association with CellTech Publications, Klamath Falls, Oregon, 1995, pp. 20–4.

Barry, W., *The Astonishing, Magnificent, Delightful Algae,* Graphic Press, Klamath Falls, Oregon, 1996, pp. 1–2.

Abrahms, K. J., *Algae to the Rescue,* Logan House, Studio City, CA, 1996, p. 7.

137. Kollman, D., *Hope Is a Molecule,* Cell Tech Publications, Klamath Falls, Oregon, 1989, pp. 2–4.

138. Personal communication between the author and scientist Dr. William Barry, author of *The Astonishing, Magnificent, Delightful Algae.*

139. Bell, L. S. and Fairchild, N. L., "Composition of algaes," *American Dietetic Association,* vol. 87, 1987, p. 341.

140. Beach, R., "Modern miracle men", 74th Congress, 2nd session US Senate Document, no. 264, June 1936, US Government Printing Office, Washington, DC, 1941, p. 1.

141. Sevilla, I. and A., *The Nicaragua Report,* Nereyda Press, Universidad Centroamericana Facultad de Ciencias Agropecuarias, Nicaragua, May 1995, p. 5.

142. Cousens, G., "Treatment of Alzheimer's disease," *Journal of Orthomolecular Medical Society,* vol. 8, nos 1 and 2, 1985, pp. 9–10.

143. Howell, E., *Enzyme Nutrition,* Avery Publishing Group, New York, p. 29.

144. Lee, L., *Earth Letter* vol. 1 no. 2, Lee Publications, Redwood City, California, 1991, p. 2.

145. Pitchford, *Healing with Whole Foods,* p. 206.

146. Ibid, p. 206.

147. Ibid, p. 195.

148. Kulvinskas, V., *Survival into the Twenty-first Century,* 21st Century Publications, Fairfield, Iowa, 1975, pp. 24–6.

149. McKeith, *The Miracle Superfood,* p. 8.

150. Boyd, D. and Baker, D., "Inhibition of the growth of the AIDs virus," *Journal of National Cancer Institute,* vol. 81, no. 8, April 1989, pp. 1254–8.

151. "Green giants—ancient algae and modern cereal grasses, spirulina: heavenly nutrient," *Delicious Magazine,* New Hope Natural Media, a division of Penton Media Inc., Boulder, Colorado, July/August 1990, pp. 34–5.

152. Boyd and Baker, "Inhibition of the growth of the AIDs virus," pp. 1254–8

153. Howell, *Enzyme Nutrition,* p. 72.

154. Pottenger, F. M., "The effect of heat processed food and metabolized vitamin D milk on the dento-facial structure of experimental animals," *American Journal of Orthodontics and Oral Surgery,* August 1946, pp. 467–85.

155. "Status of heart processing damage to protein foods," *Journal of Nutrition Review*, vol. 8, no. 7, 1950, p. 193

156. Beard, F. T. et al., "Effects of aging and cooking on the distribution of certain amino acids and nitrogen in beef muscle," *American ME Institute Foundation*, December 1953, p. 410.

157. Kulvinskas, *Survival into the 21st Century*, p. 46.

158. Cousens, *Spiritual Nutrition and The Rainbow Diet*, p. 102.

159. McCluskey, C., "The little finger test," *The Lancet*, December 1973, p. 1503.

160. Howell, *Enzyme Nutrition*, p. 78.

161. Cousens, *Spiritual Nutrition and The Rainbow Diet*, p. 99.

162. Kouchakoff, P., "The influence of cooking food on the blood formula of man," *Proceedings: First International Congress of Microbiology*, Paris, 1930, pp. 1–8.

163. Pitchford, *Healing with Whole-Foods*, p. 432.

164. Ibid, p. 429.

165. Wagner, H., "Mucopolysaccharides and the immune system," *Journal of Medical Plant Research*, vol. 1, Academic Press, London, 1985, p. 113.

166. Pitchford, *Healing with Whole Foods*, p. 467.

167. Lu, H. C., *Chinese System of Food Cures*, Sterling Publishing Co Inc., New York, 1986, pp. 141, 169.

168. Barnes, M. and Barnes, S., "The role of soy products in reducing risk of cancer," *Journal of the National Cancer Institute*, no. 83, 1991, pp. 541–6.

169. Lu, L. et al., "Soya diets and decreased risk of breast cancer," *Cancer Epidemiological Biomarkers Preview*, no. 5, 1996, pp. 63–70 and "Soy intake and risk of breast cancer in Asians and Asian Americans," *American Journal of Nutrition*, vol. 68, no. 6, 1998, p. 437.

170. Pitchford, *Healing with Whole Foods*, p. 508.

171. Balch, P., and Balch, J., *Prescription for Dietary Wellness*, Avery, New York, 1998, p. 81.

172. Yamane, Y., "The effect of spirulina on nephrotoxicity in rats," The Annual Symposium of the Pharmaceutical Society of Japan, Chiba University, Japan, April 1998.

173. Troxler, R. and Saffer, B., "Paper: Algae derived phycocanin," Association of Dental Research General Session, 1987.

174. Sano, T. and Tanaka, Y., "Effect of dried, powdered *Chlorella vulgaris* on experimental atherosclerosis and ailmentary hypercholesterolemia in cholesterol-fed rabbits," *Artery*, vol. 14, no. 2, 1987, pp. 76–84.

175. Lieber, L., "Bee propolis: the ultimate preventative medicine," *Bestways Magazine*, Nevada, 1988.

Propolis Medical Data, The Propolis Information Bureau, Louth, Lincolnshire. A compendium of some current medical data outlining the benefit of propolis. Extracts from international research papers and journals.

Wade, C., *Health from the Hive*, Keats Publishing, New Canaan, Connecticut, 1992, p. 115.

BIBLIOGRAPHY

Bartimeus, P., "Take 6 Seaweeds," *Here's Health,* December 1995.

Bartimeus, P., "Bean Power," *Here's Health,* October 1996.

Bartimeus, P., *Eating With The Seasons,* Element, Dorset, 1998.

Bradford, P. and Montse, *Cooking With Sea Vegetables,* Healing Arts Press, Vermont, 1985.

Carper, J., *Food Your Miracle Medicine,* Simon and Schuster, New York, 1993.

Chelf, V. R., *Cooking With The Right Side Of The Brain,* Avery, New York, 1991.

Cichoke, A., *Enzymes and Enzyme Therapy,* Keats Publishing, Connecticut, 1994.

Colbin, A., *Food and Healing,* Ballantine Books, New York, 1986.

Cousens, G., *Spiritual Nutrition and the Rainbow Diet,* Cassandra Press, San Rafael, CA, 1986.

Cousens, G., *Conscious Eating,* Essene Vision Books, Arizona, 1992

Foster, S., *Herbs For Your Health,* Interweave Press, Colorado, 1996.

Gage, D., *Aloe Vera,* Healing Arts Press, Vermont, 1988.

Gerras, C., *Rodale's Basic Natural Foods Cookbook,* Simon and Schuster, New York, 1984.

Goular, F. S., *Super Healing Foods,* Parker Publishing, New York, 1995.

Haas, E. M., *Staying Healthy with Nutrition,* Cassandra Press, San Rafael, CA, 1986.

Haas, E. M., *Staying Healthy with Nutrition,* Celestial Arts, California, 1992.

Heinerman, J., *Aloe Vera, Jojoba and Yucca,* Keats Publishing, Connecticut, 1982.

Holmes, P., *The Energetics of Western Herbs,* Snow Lotus Press, Colorado, 1989.

Howell, E., *Enzyme Nutrition,* Avery Publishing, New Jersey, 1985.

Ingram, C., *Self-Test Nutrition Guide*, Knowledge House, Illinois, 1994.

Kenton, L., *Passage to Power*, Vermilion, London, 1996.

Kenton, L., *The New Biogenic Diet*, Vermilion, London, 1995.

Kulvinskas, V., *Nutritional Evaluation of Sprouts and Grasses*, Omangod Press, Wethersfield, Connecticut, 1978.

Kulvinskas, V., *Survival into the 21st Century*, 21st Century Publications, Fairfield, Iowa, 1975.

Kushi, M., *The Practically Macrobiotic Cookbook*, Thorsons, London, 1987.

McKeith, G., *10 Steps To Perfect Health For All Mothers*, Lowell House (Keats Division), Los Angeles, California, 2000

McKeith, G, *The Miracle Superfood, Wild Blue-Green Algae*, Keats Publishing, Connecticut, 1998.

Meyerowitz, S., *Sprout It*, The Sprout House, Massachusetts, 1983.

Murray, M., *The Healing Power of Foods*, Prima Publishing, California, 1993.

Murray, M., and Pizzorno, J., *Encyclopedia of Natural Medicine*, Prima Health, California, 1988.

Pitchford, P., *Healing With Whole Foods*, North Atlantic Books, California, 1993.

Plaskett, L., *The Health and Medical Use of Aloe Vera*, Aloe Information Service, Cornwall, 1996.

Ridgeway, J., *Sprouting Beans and Seeds*, Century Publishing, Los Angeles, California, 1984.

Ritchason, J., *The Little Herb Encyclopedia*, Woodland Health Books, Utah, 1995.

Rogers, C., *The Women's Guide to Herbal Medicine*, Hamish Hamilton, London, 1995.

Rogers, S., *The Cure Is In The Kitchen*, Prestige Publishing, New York, 1990.

Skousen, M. B., *Aloe Vera*, Aloe Vera Research Institute, Utah, 1982.

Tenney, D., *Aloe Vera*, Woodland Publishing, Utah, 1997.

Tiwari, M., *Ayurveda—A Life Of Balance*, Healing Arts Press, Vermont, 1995.

Werbach, M., *Nutritional Influences on Illness*, Keats Publishing, New Canaan, Connecticut, 1987.

Wigmore, A., *The Hippocrates Diet*, Avery Publishing, New Jersey, 1983.

Wittenburg, M. M., *Good Food*, The Crossing Press, California, 1995.

INDEX

ABOUT THE
AUTHOR

Dr. Gillian McKeith is the internationally acclaimed clinical nutritionist and director of the renowned McKeith Clinic in London, where her extensive clientele includes professional and Olympic athletes, members of the royal family, and Hollywood stars. There is a two-year waiting list for a consultation with Dr. McKeith because of her extraordinary success in helping people to get well.

For several years Dr. McKeith was the healthy living expert for *The Joan Rivers Television Show* in the United States and the executive producer and co-host of the *Healthline Across America* radio show from New York. She presents the *Dr. Gillian McKeith's Feel Fab Forever* weekly television segment on Granada's *This Morning* television program.

Gillian holds qualifications, degrees, and a doctorate (Ph.D.) from top colleges and universities including Ivy League's University of Pennsylvania, Edinburgh University, the American College of Nutrition, the East West College of Herbalism, the Kailish Center of Oriental Medicine, and the London School of Acupuncture.

Raised in the Scottish Highlands, Gillian now travels extensively giving lectures and seminars to packed audiences. Her lifelong mission is to share her information and improve people's lives.